OXFORD MEDICAL PUBLICATIONS

Critical Care Cases

Critical Care Cases

Edited by

R. F. ARMSTRONG

Consultant in Anaesthesia and Intensive Care
University College and Middlesex Hospitals
London

and

J. B. SALMON

Consultant Physician, Intensive Care Unit
The Royal Hospital Haslar
Gosport, Hants

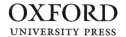

OXFORD
UNIVERSITY PRESS

OXFORD

UNIVERSITY PRESS

Great Clarendon Street, Oxford OX2 6DP

Oxford University Press is a department of the University of Oxford.
It furthers the University's objective of excellence in research, scholarship,
and education by publishing worldwide in

Oxford   New York

Athens Auckland Bangkok Bogotá Buenos Aires Calcutta
Cape Town Chennai Dar es Salaam Delhi Florence Hong Kong Istanbul
Karachi Kuala Lumpur Madrid Melbourne Mexico City Mumbai
Nairobi Paris São Paulo Singapore Taipei Tokyo Toronto Warsaw
with associated companies in Berlin Ibadan

Published in the United States
by Oxford University Press Inc., New York

First published 1997
Reprinted 2000

A catalogue record for this book is available from the British Library

Library of Congress Cataloging in Publication Data
Critical care cases / [edited by] R.F. Armstrong, J.B. Salmon
(Oxford medical publications)
Includes bibliographical references.
1. Critical care medicine—Case studies.   I. Armstrong, R. F.
(Rod F.)   II. Salmon, J. B. (Jonathan B.)   III. Series.
[DNLM: 1. Critical Care—case studies.   WX 218 C9336 1997]
RC86.7.C714   1997   616'.028—dc21   96-50462
ISBN 0 19 262584 5 (Hbk.)
ISBN 0 19 262583 7 (Pbk.)

Printed in Great Britain
on acid-free paper by
Bookcraft Ltd., Midsomer Norton, Avon

Contents

Part 5 Neurological disorder

Part 6 Metabolic

Part 7 Renal, hepatic, endocrine

Part 8 Obstetric and paediatrics

Part 9 Ethics

Preface

Intensive care overlaps most acute specialities. Its steady growth now requires an understanding of a wide range of disease processes and therapies drawn from other medical fields. At the same time there are techniques and treatment strategies which translate well from the intensive care unit to the immediate management of acutely-ill patients on general wards. However whilst most disciplines and professional examinations now demand some understanding of intensive care, opportunities for learning intensive care medicine are limited.

This problem will become more pronounced if the recommendations of the Intercollegiate Committee for Intensive Care Training are accepted and a period of time spent in intensive care becomes desirable or mandatory for junior doctors.

The aim of this book is to provide trainees with some insights into the process of intensive care. It is based on the North East Thames course, now in its seventh year. It offers a cross-section of common problems seen in intensive care, presented by clinicians working in this field. Case histories and investigations are followed by general questions and a brief discussion of the management issues. All the cases are based on real patients. It is not a substitute for clinical experience but we hope it will provide a stimulating framework for discussion and teaching.

Several aspects of the book deserve further explanation. In some of the discussions, similar points are raised: these relate mainly to management of circulation and mechanical ventilation. These two issues are so fundamental to intensive care that no discussion of an individual patient would be complete without them. Occasionally, different methods of treatment are described for similar problems. We considered editing these to provide more consistency but decided it was better to show the range of approaches used by experts in the speciality. Although underlying principles of treatment are usually similar, there are occasions where no consensus exists on the best way to reach treatment goals.

Finally, we would like to express our thanks to all our expert contributors. We hope their expertise and enthusiasm will prove contagious to those young doctors who are considering a career in this fascinating and rewarding field of medical care.

London   R.F.A.
January 1997   J.B.S.

Abbreviations

ADH	antidiuretic hormone
ALF	acute liver failure
ALT	alanine aminotransferase
ARDS	acute respiratory distress syndrome
ARF	acute renal failure
AST	aspartate aminotransferase
ATN	acute tubular necrosis
BE	base excess
CBF	cerebral blood flow
Cdyn	dynamic compliance
CFT	complement fixation test
CI	cardiac index
CIN	critical illness neuropathy
CK	creatine kinase
COPD	chronic obstructive pulmonary disease
CPAP	continuous positive airway pressure
CPP	cerebral perfusion pressure
CSF	cerebrospinal fluid
CT	computed tomography
CVP	central venous pressure
DIC	disseminated intravascular coagulation
ELISA	enzyme linked immunosorbent assay
ERCP	endoscopic retrograde cholangiopancreatography
ETT	endotracheal tube
FDPs	fibrinogen degradation products
FFP	fresh frozen plasma
f/Vt	ratio of breathing frequency to tidal volume
GCS	Glasgow coma score
GFR	glomerular filtration rate
HBO	hyperbaric oxygen
HIV	human immunodeficiency virus
ICP	intracranial pressure
I:E	inspiration:expiration
IFAT	immunofluorescent antibody test
IgM	immunoglobulin M
IPPV	intermittent positive pressure ventilation
IRV	inverse ratio ventilation
LDH	lactate dehydrogenase
LOI	lactate oxygen index
MAP	mean arterial pressure
MI	myocardial infarction
MPAP	mean pulmonary artery pressure
MRI	magnetic resonance imaging

NSAIDS	non-steroidal anti-inflammatory drugs
PAC	pulmonary artery catheter
PAOP	pulmonary artery occlusion pressure
Paw	airway pressure
PCP	*Pneumocystis carinii* pneumonia
PCR	polymerase chain reaction
PE	pulmonary embolus
PEEP	positive end-expiratory pressure
PCV	pressure control ventilation
PVR	pulmonary vascular resistance
REM	rapid eye movement
RMAT	rapid micro agglutination test
SIMV	synchronized intermittent mandatory ventilation
SVR	systemic vascular resistance
TBSA	total body surface area
TNF	tumour necrosis factor
TOE	transoesophageal echocardiography
VC	vital capacity
Vt	tidal volume
WIF	whole inclusion immunofluorescence (test)

Normal values

MEASURED CARDIOVASCULAR VARIABLES

Cardiac output (CO)	4–6 L/min
Stroke volume (SV)	70–100 ml
Right atrial pressure (RAP)	0–5 mmHg
Right ventricular pressure (RVP)	20–25/0–5 mmHg
Pulmonary artery pressure (PAP)	20–25/10–15 mmHg
Pulmonary artery occlusion pressure (PAOP)	6–12 mmHg
Mixed venous oxygen saturation (SvO_2)	70–75%

DERIVED CARDIOVASCULAR VARIABLES

Cardiac index (CI):	$\dfrac{CO}{\text{Body surface area}}$	2.5–3.5 L/min/m^2
Stroke index (SVI):	$\dfrac{SV}{\text{Body surface area}}$	40–60 ml/m^2
Systemic vascular resistance (SVR):	$\dfrac{(MAP - RAP) \times 79.9}{CO}$	960–1400 dyn/sec/cm^{-5}
Pulmonary vascular resistance (PVR):	$\dfrac{(MAP - PAWP) \times 79.9}{CO}$	25–125 dyn/sec/cm^{-5}
Left ventricular stroke work index (LVSWI):	$(MAP - PAWP) \times SVI \times 0.0136$	44–68 g-m/m^2/beat
Right ventricular stroke work index (RVSWI):	$(MPAP - RAP) \times SVI \times 0.0136$	4–8 g-m/m^2/beat
Oxygen delivery (DO_2)	$0.134 \times CO \times Hb \times SaO_2$	950–1300 ml/min
Oxygen consumption (VO_2)	$0.134 \times CO \times (Hb \times SaO_2 - Hb \times SvO_2)$	180–320 ml/min

ARTERIAL BLOOD GASES

PaO_2	12.5 kPa (age 20 yr) to 10.8 kPa (60–69 yr)
$PaCO_2$	5.3 kPa
pH	7.36–7.44
HCO_3	22–26 mmol/l
BE	−2.4 to +2.2

Part 1 Respiratory

1.1 ACUTE RESPIRATORY FAILURE

R. F. ARMSTRONG FRCA

Consultant in Anaesthesia and Intensive Care
Middlesex Hospital
UCL
London

CASE HISTORY

A 60-year-old male patient was admitted with a 5-day history of malaise, cough with purulent sputum, and increasing breathlessness.

EXAMINATION FINDINGS

Central cyanosis; dyspnoea; using accessory muscles of respiration; tongue dry; temperature 38°C; pulse irregular 140/min. Blood pressure (BP) 80/60 mmHg; respiratory rate 40/min. Chest dull to percussion on left with reduced air entry. Central venous pressure (CVP) 0 mmHg. Chest X-ray revealed opacification of the whole of the left lung.

INVESTIGATIONS

Biochemistry		Arterial blood gases (FiO2 0.6)	
Sodium	150 mmol/l	PaO_2	13.0 kPa
Potassium	4.8 mmol/l	$PaCO_2$	9.6 kPa
Creatinine	150 μmol/l	pH	7.10
Chloride	108 mmol/l	HCO_3	24 mmol/l
Bicarbonate	30 mmol/l	BE	0 mmol/l
Urea	20 mmol/l	SaO_2	100%

DISCUSS MANAGEMENT AND TREATMENT

He is in respiratory failure on several counts. He has a respiratory rate well over 30/min, a level at which respiratory work becomes excessive. He is using his accessory muscles of respiration. The PaO_2 of 13 kPa is much lower than it should be (he is on 60% oxygen) as is clear from a consideration of the simplified air equation. This shows that on an FiO_2 of 0.6 and with a $PaCO_2$ of 9.6 kPa, this patient's PaO_2 should be approximately 43 kPa.

e.g. PAO_2 = FiO_2 (Pb $-PH_2O$) $-$ $PaCO_2$/RQ
     PAO_2 = 0.6 (100 $-$ 6) $-$ 9.6/0.8
     PAO_2 = 54 $-$ 12 = 43 kPa

Where PAO_2 = partial pressure of alveolar oxygen; FiO_2 = fractional inspired oxygen concentration; Pb = barometric pressure; PH_2O = partial pressure of water vapour; $PaCO_2$ = partial pressure of arterial carbon dioxide; RQ = respiratory quotient. PaO_2 =partial pressure of arterial oxygen.

A PAO_2 of 43 kPa should result in a slightly lower PaO_2 (about 40 kPa) due to the presence of a small degree of shunt in the normal patient (1–4% of the cardiac output).

The SaO_2 of 100% is misleadingly good. From the dissociation curve it is clear that once the patient achieves any PaO_2 above 12 kPa then the haemoglobin will be fully saturated. However, whilst oxygen content is admittedly satisfactory, consideration of the PaO_2 demonstrates a serious respiratory disorder. His PaO_2 is in fact less than one-third what it should be. There is also a severe respiratory acidosis for which there has not yet been adequate renal compensation.

This picture suggests acute respiratory deterioration and given that the pH is now below 7.2 he needs urgent respiratory support.

A review of the electrolyte measurements shows an element of renal failure, probably due to dehydration. This is supported by the raised sodium and low CVP. He may well be hypovolaemic and if time allows, judicious fluid replacement is indicated using a colloid fluid given in repeated small aliquots. CVP and BP should be reviewed after each fluid challenge to determine whether more will be required. In the absence of a satisfactory response, left-sided filling pressures should be assessed, though this will have to wait until respiratory support has been initiated.

The insertion of an arterial line will facilitate management by allowing beat-to-beat monitoring of BP during resuscitation.

Once hypovolaemia is reversed the patient needs intubation and ventilating. After preoxygenation, a rapid sequence induction using etomidate and a short-acting muscle relaxant is probably the safest combination, with continuous monitoring of the common variables. Suxamethonium should be avoided in the presence of hyperkalaemia, burns, neuropathy/paralysis, and abdominal sepsis. Cricoid pressure and available suction is important.

All resuscitation drugs, especially atropine and 10 ml of 1:10 000 adrenaline, should be readily available. Whilst the patient is lying flat for intubation this is a good opportunity for central line insertion, pulmonary artery catheterization if not already done, and nasogastric tube insertion. All can then be assessed by one X-ray.

The patient was ventilated, treated with antibiotics, and given appropriate fluids. Atrial fibrillation reverted to sinus rhythm after rehydration. Slow improvement resulted in weaning after 2 weeks intensive care.

KEY POINTS

1. When assessing respiratory function, compare actual PaO_2 with predicted PaO_2, calculated by observation of the FiO_2 and use of the simplified alveolar air equation.
2. Ventilation should be considered:
   (a) on clinical grounds (ie use of accessory muscles)
   (b) when the respiratory rate is > 30/min
   (c) when the $PaCO_2$ is high enough to lower the pH below 7.2
   (d) when the PaO_2 is less than one-third what it should be.
3. Patients with significant impairment of respiratory function may have a normal oxygen saturation if on oxygen therapy.

FURTHER READING

Armstrong, R. F. (1994) The interpretation of arterial blood gases. *Curr. Anaes. Crit. Care*, 5, 74–80.

Schuster, D. P. (1990) A physiological approach to initiating, maintaining, and withdrawing mechanical ventilatory support during acute respiratory failure. *Am. J. Med.* 88, 268–78.

Tremper, K. K. and Barker, S. J. (1989) Pulse oximetry. *Anesthesiology*, 70, 98–108.

NOTES

1.2 CHRONIC RESPIRATORY FAILURE

ANITA SIMONDS MD FRCP
Consultant Physician
The Royal Brompton Hospital
London

CASE HISTORY

A 54-year-old delivery man was admitted to a medical ward with a 3-day history of breathlessness, wheeze, and cough with purulent sputum. He had smoked 25 cigarettes a day for 40 years, but had never previously been hospitalized for a respiratory problem. His only regular medication was inhaled salbutamol. Exercise tolerance was reported by his family to be around 400 m on the flat until this current episode.

EXAMINATION FINDINGS

Dyspnoeic at rest, and cyanosed, with a heart rate of 120/min. Chest hyperinflated with widespread inspiratory and expiratory wheeze, and generalized poor air entry.

INVESTIGATIONS

Chest X-ray: hyperinflated, emphysematous lung fields, no pneumothorax.
ECG: Sinus tachycardia, P-pulmonale
Peak flow: 60 l/min
FEV_1/FVC: 500 / 1900 ml

Arterial blood gases

FiO_2 0.21
PaO_2 5.4 kPa
$PaCO_2$ 8.1 kPa
pH 7.27
HCO_3 34 mmol/l

The patient was treated intensively with controlled oxygen therapy, nebulized bronchodilators, hydrocortisone, antibiotics, and physiotherapy to aid sputum clearance. Despite this, over the next few hours he becam~

progressively more exhausted and agitated. Arterial blood gas tensions (FiO_2 0.24) showed PaO_2 6.7 kPa, $PaCO_2$ 10.4 kPa, pH 7.22. In view of this deterioration he was transferred electively to the intensive care unit, intubated, and ventilated. Over the next 36 hours sputum cleared and wheeze settled. The patient was extubated and returned to a general ward. However, the following night he again became confused and dyspnoeic. Repeat arterial blood gas testing showed that $PaCO_2$ had risen from 7.0 kPa earlier in the day to 13.3 kPa on a FiO_2 of 0.24. He was reintubated and intermittent positive pressure ventilation (IPPV) reinstituted. Over the next two weeks repeated attempts at weaning failed and a tracheostomy was performed. Despite being able to breathe spontaneously for 30 minutes on low levels of inspiratory pressure support, during trials of spontaneous ventilation the patient rapidly developed tachypnoea accompanied by bronchospasm, panic, and a rise in $PaCO_2$.

DESCRIBE THE FURTHER MANAGEMENT OF WEANING IN THIS PATIENT

The patient has clinical and radiological features of severe chronic obstructive pulmonary disease (COPD). The arterial blood gas tensions on admission demonstrate acute on chronic type II respiratory failure. The patient was intubated because of progressive acidosis and uncontrolled hypercapnia while receiving controlled oxygen therapy.

Weaning problems occur in around 20% of patients receiving IPPV, those with chronic lung disease being at particular risk. Here the return to spontaneous ventilation is hindered by an imbalance between the load placed on the respiratory system, the capacity of the thoracic pump to compensate for added load, and central respiratory drive. In the COPD patient receiving IPPV, the load on the respiratory system is increased by airflow obstruction (bronchospasm, mucus plugging, resistance of the endotracheal tube and ventilatory circuit), hyperinflation, and positive end-expiratory pressure (intrinsic PEEP).

The capacity of the respiratory muscles to compensate for this added load is compromised by hypercapnia, hypoxaemia, acidosis, malnutrition, and metabolic disarray, including hypophosphataemia and hypomagnesaemia. Doxapram is often used to stimulate central drive but in many COPD patients drive is normal or even increased during an exacerbation. Even if the balance between load and capacity is sustained when the patient is awake, respiration during sleep poses a particular challenge for individuals with chronic lung disease as intercostal muscle activity wanes and ventilatory responses to hypercapnia and hypoxia reach a nadir in rapid eye movement (REM) sleep.

Once the precipitating event has resolved (e.g. infection), the approach to weaning should focus on minimizing load and maximizing ventilatory capacity. Optimization of treatment for airflow obstruction should include nebulized bronchodilator, steroids to reduce airway inflammation, humidification and physiotherapy to clear secretions. Full patency of an endotracheal tube or tracheostomy of adequate calibre should be confirmed and steps taken to investigate for left and right ventricular dysfunction, treating this where necessary. Hyperinflation should be avoided.

Numerous ventilatory techniques have been advocated to improve the chances of weaning success, including synchronized intermittent mandatory ventilation (SIMV), inspiratory pressure support, and continuous positive airway pressure (CPAP).

However, where these techniques fail, as in this case, it is worth considering non-invasive positive pressure ventilation via a nasal or full facemask. This has the advantage of allowing the extubated patient to eat, drink, and communicate normally while improving mobilization, and removes the risks accompanying intubation such as nosocomial infection, tracheal stenosis, etc. The level of ventilatory support can be gradually tailed off depending on the patient's progress. In this case, nasal mask ventilation was initiated using a pressure support non-invasive ventilator

(BiPAP, Respironics Ltd.) with the tracheostomy cuff deflated and stoma occluded. After successful mask ventilation overnight, the tracheostomy was removed and the patient maintained on nasal ventilation initially for 16 hours a day. Within 4 days it was possible to reduce ventilatory support to night-time use only.

Night-time ventilation was discontinued after a further week when overnight monitoring showed satisfactory control of SpO_2 and $PaCO_2$ during sleep. Arterial blood gases (FiO_2 0.21) on discharge were PaO_2 7.9 kPa, $PaCO_2$ 6.3 kPa, HCO_3 27 mmol/l.

Non-invasive mask ventilation may be useful in averting the need for intubation and conventional ventilation in some patients. Recent controlled studies have shown that non-invasive mask ventilation can reduce intubation rate, shorten hospital stay, and decrease in-hospital mortality in selected COPD patients with a hypercapnic exacerbation. Non-invasive ventilation should therefore be considered in COPD patients with acute hypercapnic decompensation who fail to respond to conventional therapeutic measures.

KEY POINTS

1. Weaning from positive pressure ventilation may be achieved by minimizing load and maximizing ventilatory capacity.
2. Non-invasive positive pressure ventilation by nasal mask or face mask is a useful alternative when weaning difficulties are encountered.

FURTHER READING

Bott, J., Carroll, M., Conway, J. H., et al. (1993) Randomised controlled trial of nasal ventilation in acute ventilatory failure due to chronic obstructive airways disease. Lancet, 341, 1555–7.

Brochard, L., Mancebo, J., Wysocki, M., et al. (1995) Non-invasive ventilation for acute exacerbations of chronic obstructive pulmonary disease. N. Engl. J. Med., 333, 817–22.

Goldstone, J. and Moxham, J. (1994) Weaning from mechanical ventilation. In (ed. J. Goldstone and J. Moxham) Assisted ventilation, pp. 57–79. BMJ Publishing Group, London.

Udwadia, Z., Santis, G. K., Steven, M. H., and Simonds, A. K. (1992) Nasal ventilation to facilitate weaning in patients with chronic resp. insufficiency. Thorax, 47, 715–18.

1.3 ASTHMA

BRIAN F. KEOGH FRCA
Consultant in Anaesthesia and Intensive Care
Royal Brompton Hospital
London

CASE HISTORY

An 18-year-old male suffered a severe asthma attack at home in association with a recent upper respiratory tract infection. On arrival in the A&E department, the ambulance officers reported that the patient was initially conscious but unable to speak and had rapidly become unresponsive during transfer. On initial assessment, despite mask oxygen, SpO_2 was 65% and the patient essentially apnoeic in gross hyperinflation. The patient was immediately intubated by A&E staff and manually ventilated with FiO_2 1.0. Nebulized salbutamol was commenced and intravenous hydrocortisone 200 mg administered.

The intensive care team were immediately called. Attempts to manually hyperventilate the patient had proven extremely difficult, but SpO_2 had increased to 88%.

EXAMINATION FINDINGS

On examination the chest was silent, grossly hyperinflated, and the patient suffused with prominent external jugular veins. Heart rate was 145/min, automated BP recording was impossible, peripheral pulses were absent, and carotid pulsation could just be determined. Peripheral SpO_2 measurements could no longer be recorded.

INVESTIGATIONS

Biochemistry		Arterial blood gases	
Sodium	147 mmol/l	pH	6.8
Potassium	3.0 mmol/l	$PaCO_2$	14.0 kPa
Blood sugar	14 mmol/l	PaO_2	9.0 kPa
Haemoglobin (Hb)	18.8 g/dl	HCO_3	16 mmol/l
		BE	−8 mmol/l

The family reported subsequently that the patient was a mild asthmatic, took nebulized salbutamol only occasionally when he felt wheezy, and was otherwise fit. They reported that he had had 'the flu' for two days and had been increasingly unwell and complaining of breathlessness during the previous 8 hours.

DISCUSS MANAGEMENT AND TREATMENT

Immediate problems are extreme hyperinflation, haemodynamic depression, and hypovolaemia. Low tidal volume (6–8ml/kg) and low frequency (5–10/min) manual ventilation with long expiratory times are indicated, initially with paralysis.

Oxygenation and haemodynamic resuscitation are primary concerns and carbon dioxide clearance a secondary issue. Rapid colloid infusion, at least 20 ml/kg, is necessary to support intravascular volume (CVP measurements are unreliable). No immediate improvement mandates inotropic support – adrenaline 10–50 μg bolus if necessary, and by infusion at 0.1–0.3 μg/kg/min (despite the tachycardia) in view of additional bronchodilator properties.

Consider decreasing gas trapping by (i) a period of 20–30 seconds of expiratory apnoea (disconnect completely from ventilation); or (ii) external chest compression: forcible deflation by rib compression or by 'bear hug' manoeuvre.

Add intravenous bronchodilators; salbutamol or aminophylline. In this case aminophylline was added to adrenaline as previous theophylline therapy was not an issue. In a less extreme case, salbutamol would have been preferred to adrenaline.

Transfer to ICU when stable. Continue support as above. Ventilation by low morbidity approach – rate 6–10 per minute, long expiratory time, and tidal volumes of 5–10 ml/kg, avoiding high peak pressures and dynamic hyperinflation. Accept profound hypercarbia ($PaCO_2$ 12–18 kPa) in initial stages if necessary.

Emphasis of therapy should be on cardiovascular stability. Correct hypokalaemia if persistent. Add isoflurane (1–3%) via circuit, nebulized ipratropium bromide, and budesonide and continue high dose intravenous steroids. Titration of external PEEP to influence small airway closure may be applied but only in pressure limited systems. Regular instillation of saline aliquots will mobilize mucous plugs. Bronchoscopy +/- lavage is of limited benefit.

Consider ketamine infusion (10–80 μg/kg/min), intravenous magnesium sulphate (recent report of high dose 10–20 g i.v. over one hour), and ventilation with Heliox. Extracorporeal support is an absolute last resort, to be instituted on the basis of refractory circulatory failure rather than on gas exchange criteria.

Acute asphyxic asthma often responds quickly and requires a short ventilation time. Normal blood gases were achieved after 48 hours and extubation at 96 hours. The patient is poorly compliant, has now been lost to follow-up, and is at risk of further similar episodes.

KEY POINTS

1. Ventilation mode. The ideal ventilator for asthma provides independent control of inspiratory flow rate and inspiration:expiration (I:E) ratio with both pressure and volume limitation. The author prefers time-cycled, pressure-controlled mode to a maximum of 50 cmH$_2$0 (or less if possible) with a volume limit – to prevent iatrogenic overinflation in pressure control mode when airways resistance falls. Volume-cycled systems remain popular but provide less flexibility and a greater potential for both barotrauma and haemodynamic depression.

2. Sodium bicarbonate (NaHCO$_3$) therapy for the initial metabolic acidosis and to increase the pH in the presence of profound hypercarbia is very controversial. The author believes that NaHCO$_3$ should be avoided in view of its carbon dioxide generation – the initial metabolic acidosis is best treated with appropriate haemodynamic support and longer-term respiratory acidosis is well-tolerated. If NaHCO$_3$ is used it must be administered by very slow infusion.

3. Neuromuscular blockade. The combination of neuromuscular blockers (including atracurium) and high-dose corticosteroids may be associated with a severe myopathy. Although usually indicated in the acute phase, paralysis should be limited, if possible, during ongoing therapy.

FURTHER READING

Darioli, R. and Perret, C. (1984) Mechanical controlled hypoventilation in status asthmaticus. *Am. Rev. Resp. Dis.*, 129, 385–7.

Fisher, M. M., Bowey, C. J., and Ladd-Hudson, K. (1989) External chest compression in acute asthma: a preliminary study. *Crit. Care Med.*, 17, 686–7.

Sydow, M., Crozier, T. A., Zielmann, S., Radke, J., and Burchardi, H. (1993) High-dose intravenous magnesium sulfate in the management of life-threatening status asthmaticus. *Intensive Care Med.*, 19, 467–71.

NOTES

1.4 ACUTE RESPIRATORY DISTRESS SYNDROME (ARDS)

T. W. Evans MD FRCP PhD
Professor of Intensive Care Medicine
R. Sayeed FRCS
National Heart and Lung Institute
Royal Brompton Hospital
London

CASE HISTORY

A 26-year-old woman approaching term during her first pregnancy developed a widespread vesicular rash with associated dyspnoea of effort. Chest radiography revealed bilateral reticular shadowing. She was admitted to ITU because of refractory hypoxaemia, where a clinical diagnosis of varicella pneumonitis was made, and she proceeded to an emergency Caesarean section.

Over the next two weeks she required mechanical ventilatory support with progressively increasing concentrations of inspired oxygen and minute volume requirement to maintain acceptable arterial gas tensions. Her chest radiograph showed diffuse, bilateral alveolar shadowing. She became pyrexial (38.6°C) and her urine output fell to 20 ml/hour.

INVESTIGATIONS

Biochemistry

Sodium	138 mmol/l
Potassium	5.2 mmol/l
Urea	25 mmol/l
Creatinine	300 μmol/l
Hb	10.0 g/dl
WCC	18×10^9/l
Platelets	100×10^9/l

Arterial blood gases (FiO$_2$ 1.0)

PaO$_2$	7.5 kPa
PaCO$_2$	8.0 kPa
pH	7.26
SaO$_2$	88%

Haemodynamics

MAP	72 mmHg
PAOP	15 mmHg
SVR	720 dyne-sec/cm^{-5}
CO	6.0 L/min
MPAP	45 mmHg

RAP   18 mmHg
PVR   400 dyne-sec/cm^{-5}
HR   120/min

Where MAP = mean arterial pressure; PAOP = pulmonary artery occlusion pressure; SVR = systemic vascular resistance; CO = cardiac output; MPAP = mean pulmonary arterial pressure; RAP = right atrial pressure; PVR = pulmonary vascular resistance; HR = heart rate.

DISCUSS MANAGEMENT AND TREATMENT

This patient has developed the acute respiratory distress syndrome (ARDS) with refractory hypoxaemia ($PaO_2/FiO_2 < 26$), bilateral infiltrates on chest radiography and a PAOP < 18mmHg. ARDS is associated with a range of serious pulmonary and non-pulmonary clinical conditions. Radiographic evidence of widespread alveolar and interstitial oedema develops, resulting from increased pulmonary microvascular permeability.

ARDS probably represents only the pulmonary manifestation of a panendothelial insult which may be responsible for the development of the multisystem organ failure that often complicates the syndrome and accounts for the high associated mortality (40–80% depending upon the precipitating condition). To date, treatment remains supportive. In this case, the management problems are as follows:

1. **Refractory hypoxaemia.** The aim of mechanical ventilation in ARDS is to achieve adequate oxygenation without exacerbating the underlying lung injury. The preferred mode is probably pressure-controlled inverse ratio ventilation (PC-IRV) with low minute volumes and 'permissive' hypercapnia. In theory, the inverse I:E ratio should promote alveolar stability and the peak airway pressure limit reduce the risk of barotrauma, although controlled, prospective trials are lacking.
2. **Pulmonary hypertension.** A raised PVR (normal < 160 dyne-sec/cm^5) is associated with poor prognosis in ARDS. Secondly, abnormalities of ventilation: perfusion (V/Q) matching may account for the refractory hypoxaemia that characterizes the condition. Prostacyclin or nitric oxide (NO) administered by nebulization/inhalation selectively reduce PVR and decrease/shunt fraction by recruiting blood to ventilated alveolar units, producing sustained improvements in pulmonary haemodynamics and gas exchange.
3. **Acute renal failure.** Acute renal failure with fluid overload is shown here by abnormal electrolytes and high-filling pressures: although the pulmonary artery occlusion pressure (PAOP) was 15 mmHg, this may be high in patients with low plasma oncotic pressures. Here, the albumin was only 25 g/l, increasing the relative contribution of hydrostatic pressure to pulmonary oedema formation. At least in the short term, a negative fluid balance would be desirable, with strict review of drug infusions, feed, and maintenance fluids. To this end, continuous venovenous haemofiltration should be instigated which would also address the associated acidosis and hyperkalaemia. Circulatory support can be provided using inotropes. Renal-dose dopamine may preserve renal perfusion.
4. **Cardiovascular instability.** The cardiac output is lower than expected, indicating a degree of myocardial dysfunction and her SVR is low (both attributable to systemic sepsis). A noradrenaline infusion might be needed to raise peripheral vascular resistance to maintain main arterial pressure (MAP) particularly if aggressive fluid removal is contemplated

(see 3). Intravenous adrenaline may also be required if the (relatively) low CO leads to impaired tissue perfusion. This is shown by clinical assessment and by the development of a high lactate, or mixed venous oxygen saturation less than 60%.

5. **Infection.** The high WCC, low SVR, and pyrexia, suggest supra-added infection. Broad-spectrum antibiotics should be commenced after appropriate cultures. The diagnosis of varicella pneumonitis needs to be confirmed and intravenous acyclovir continued beyond the customary 2 weeks.

6. **Haematological problems.** Thrombocytopenia may herald the development of disseminated intravascular coagulation. A full clotting screen, including cross-linked fibrin degradation products, is needed. Appropriate treatment includes fresh frozen plasma (FFP) and platelet infusions and possibly a heparin infusion for any clotting tendency. The patient was also anaemic, but only a haemoglobin consistently below 10 g/dl would normally merit transfusion.

7. **Other measures.** The FiO$_2$ should be kept as low as possible commensurate with an oxygen delivery of 330 ml/min/m^2 to avoid oxygen toxicity. Extracorporeal support techniques are not indicated in general terms. In patients in whom computed tomography (CT scanning) reveals sparing of non-dependent parts of the lung, nursing in the prone position may markedly improve V/Q matching and therefore oxygenation. Steroid therapy may be indicated in individual cases with isolated respiratory failure, in whom infection has been excluded, but this remains contentious.

FURTHER READING

Bernard, G., Artigas, A., Brigham, K., et al. (1994) The American–European consensus conference on ARDS. *Am. J. Respir. Crit. Care Med.*, 149, 818–24.

Braude, S., Haslam, P., Hughes, D., Macnaughton, P. D. and Evans, T. W. (1992) 'Chronic' adult respiratory distress syndrome – a role for corticosteroids? *Crit. Care Med.*, 20, 1187–90.

Keogh, B. F. and Evans, T. W. (1991) Extracorporeal membrane oxygenation: a breath of fresh air or yesterday's therapy? *Thorax*, 46, 692–4.

Macnaughton, P. D. and Evans, T. W. (1992) Adult respiratory distress syndrome. *Lancet*, 339, 469–72.

1.5 VENTILATOR MANAGEMENT

C. FERGUSON FRCA

Consultant and Honorary Senior Lecturer
Intensive Care Unit
St Bartholomew's Hospital
London

CASE HISTORY

A 38-year-old female patient who had taken an overdose of tricyclic antidepressants presented with tachyarrythmias and convulsions having been transferred intubated from another hospital.

INVESTIGATIONS

Arterial blood gases on arrival (FiO$_2$ 0.4)

PaO$_2$	30.8 kPa
PaCO$_2$	4.7 kPa
BE	5 mmols/l

Deliberate hyperventilation was instituted and subsequent gases (FiO$_2$ 0.3) were PaO$_2$ 15.2 kPa, PaCO$_2$ 4.07 kPa, base excess 1.6 mmols/l. Her fits were eventually controlled with a thiopentone infusion and the tachyarrythmias resolved after alkalinization with large doses of sodium bicarbonate. Subsequently however she developed adult respiratory distress syndrome and 36 hours later blood gases had deteriorated to PaO$_2$ 6.5 kPa, PaCO$_2$ 6.7 kPa (FiO$_2$ 0.8).

At this stage she was receiving volume-controlled intermittent positive pressure ventilation with 10 cmH$_2$O PEEP, a rate of 10 breaths per minute, and a tidal volume of 700 ml. Peak airway pressure was 46 cmH$_2$O. Immediate increase of the FiO$_2$ to 1.0 resulted in a PaO$_2$ of 7.2 kPa.

DISCUSS MANAGEMENT AND TREATMENT

There are three problems involved in the ventilation of this patient – hypoxaemia, high airway pressures, and inadequate carbon dioxide clearance. The high pressures reflect the severity of the lung injury and present a constant threat of barotrauma producing a pneumothorax. Any increase in PEEP therefore should be judicious and can be estimated from the inflection point on a pressure volume curve constructed for this patient's lungs.

Oxygenation may be further improved by inverse ratio ventilation (IRV), that is prolonging inspiratory time to reverse the conventional I:E ratio so that inspiration is longer than expiration. This may maintain gas exchange at lower levels of PEEP, recruit slow alveoli, and avoid overdistension of the normal alveoli. IRV may be administered by volume-controlled or pressure-controlled ventilation. The advantage of the latter is that peak pressure is fixed at the level set on the ventilator. The concomitant disadvantage is that tidal volume then becomes a function of the patient's respiratory mechanics and minute volume cannot be prescribed. The patient was transferred to pressure controlled IRV. Initial PEEP of 10 cmH$_2$O resulted in immediate desaturation, but at PEEP of 15 cmH$_2$O, tidal volume 540 ml, pressure control of 30 cmH$_2$O, FiO$_2$ of 1.0, respiratory rate of 10/min., and an I:E ratio of 2:1, the PaO$_2$ was 8.5 kPa and the PaCO$_2$ 4.84 kPa. Thus oxygenation was improved with no additional pressure cost, and tidal volume kept low to avoid volutrauma – overdistension of compliant units of the lung.

The patient continued to improve over the next day whilst efforts were made to achieve a negative fluid balance without jeopardizing oxygen delivery and organ perfusion. Attempts to reduce the driving pressure were unsuccessful in that they led to immediate desaturation.

Thirty-six hours later, on the same ventilator settings, apart from a rate increase to 12, the PaO$_2$ had improved to 23.4 kPa with a PaCO$_2$ of 7.5 kPa. However, the tidal volume had fallen to 440 ml reflecting the ongoing lung injury.

The FiO$_2$ could now be reduced to 0.8 with maintenance of adequate oxygenation. However, the patient's condition subsequently deteriorated with the onset of systemic sepsis and haemodynamic instability. Oxygenation could not be maintained even with an increase of FiO$_2$ to 1.0. Use of the prone position was contraindicated by the difficulty in maintaining blood pressure and altering the I:E ratio to 4:1 only resulted in transient improvement. Septic shock ensued and the patient died with terminal vasoplegia.

KEY POINTS

1. Pressure-controlled inverse ratio ventilation can improve oxygenation and reduce ventilator-related lung damage.
2. Volume trauma should be avoided.
3. The cost of improved oxygenation may include respiratory acidosis (raised $PaCO_2$) and the need for paralysis and deep sedation.
4. The effects of altering I:E ratio and thus the specific ratio required are unpredictable and must be titrated individually.
5. Use of the prone position may result in improvement in blood gases.
6. Current management of ARDS includes 'drying out' the patient but without jeopardizing oxygen flow to other organ systems.
7. There is no place for steroids in early ARDS but anecdotal evidence suggests they may have a place at 7–10 days during the fibro-proliferative stage of lung damage.

FURTHER READING

Kollef, M. H. and Schuster, D. P. (1995) The acute respiratory distress syndrome. *N. Engl. J. Med.*, **332**, 27–34.

Marcy, T. W. and Marini, J. J. (1991) Inverse ratio ventilation in ARDS: rationale and implementation. *Chest*, **100**, 494–504.

Slutsky, A. S. (1994) Consensus conference on mechanical ventilation. Part 2. *Intensive Care Med.*, **20**, 150–62.

Tuxen, D. V. (1994) Permissive hypercapnic ventilation. *Am. J. Respir. Crit. Care Med.*, **150**, 870–4.

NOTES

1.6 VENTILATOR MANAGEMENT

GEORGE G. COLLEE FRCA
Consultant in Anaesthesia and Intensive Care
Intensive Care Unit
The Royal Free Hospital
London

CASE HISTORY

A 45-year-old, 75 kg man was admitted to hospital with severe acute pancreatitis. Two days after admission he developed respiratory failure requiring mechanical ventilation on the intensive care unit. Over the course of the next 3 days his pulmonary function continued to deteriorate.

EXAMINATION FINDINGS

Sedated with midazolam and fentanyl but rousable to noxious stimuli. Hourly urine volumes 20 ml/hr; temperature 38.5°C; BP 95/50 mmHg. Abdomen distended, tympanitic, no bowel sounds. Large gastric aspirates via NG tube.

INVESTIGATIONS

Biochemistry

Urea	18 mmol/l
Creatinine	150 μmol/l
Sodium	135 mmol/l
Potassium	4.0 mmol/l
Hb	11 g/dl
WCC	$23 \times 10^9/l$
Platelets	$70 \times 10^9/l$

Arterial blood gases (FiO$_2$ 0.8)

PaO_2	8.2 kPa
$PaCO_2$	4.2 kPa
pH	7.46
HCO_3	22 mmol/l
SaO_2	88%

Chest X-ray: diffuse patchy opacification throughout both lungs consistent with ARDS.

Ventilation

SIMV	12/min
Vt	800 ml
I:E ratio	1:2
Paw	35 cmH$_2$0
PEEP	5 cmH$_2$0

DISCUSS MANAGEMENT AND TREATMENT

To control his fever, reduce oxygen consumption, and improve ventilation this man should be sedated and paralysed. The oliguria and uraemia may be indicative of hypovolaemia and before any changes are made to the level of PEEP or mode of ventilation, an intravenous fluid volume challenge should be performed. A pulmonary artery catheter would be useful to optimize his cardiac function in these circumstances.

A SpO_2 > 90% should be achieved to ensure an adequate oxygen content in the arterial blood.

The PEEP of 5 cmH_2O is low. Inspired oxygen concentrations above 60% may be associated with oxygen toxicity. Thus in order to reduce FiO_2 the PEEP should be increased in increments of 2.5–5 cmH_2O towards a maximum of 10–12.5 cmH_2O, looking for an improvement in PaO_2 and in total thoracic compliance. Changes in PEEP may take about 2 hours to be effective. Improvements in compliance are implied by finding a smaller increment rise in plateau pressure than the increment rise in PEEP. In ventilators which incorporate graphics it may be useful to look for the inflexion point on the inspiratory limb of the pressure volume loop as a guide to the best PEEP level. If the stroke volume falls on introduction of PEEP, consider further volume loading.

The $PaCO_2$ is unnecessarily low. The minute ventilation should be decreased, allowing the carbon dioxide level to rise – so-called 'permissive hypercapnia'. Reducing intrathoracic pressures reduces barotrauma. At the same time, a reduction of the tidal volume can prevent volutrauma.

Extending the inspiratory time and therefore using higher I:E ratios (e.g. 1:1, 2:1) may further improve the distribution of ventilation. In volume-controlled ventilation this is best achieved by reducing the respiratory rate and/or tidal volume, adding an end-inspiratory pause, and shortening the expiratory time. High-peak inspiratory pressures can be avoided by reducing the inspiratory flow rate, though this will prolong the inspiratory phase. Beware of gas trapping.

Some ventilators include the facilities for pressure control ventilation (PCV) and IRV. In PCV the inspiratory pressure can be limited in order to prevent volutrauma. Prolonging the inspiratory time may allow better ventilation of slow-filling units with recruitment of previously hypoventilated lung. The shortened expiratory phase may produce intrinsic PEEP in slow-emptying units of lung with recruitment of atelectatic regions. It is dangerous to manipulate the I:E ratio without closely monitoring the patient for gas trapping.

Patients who have been nursed supine for prolonged periods develop pulmonary collapse in dependent areas of lung. These changes can be minimized by regular turning. Transient improvement in gas exchange can be achieved by turning the patient prone, allowing re-expansion of previously collapsed dependent areas.

KEY POINTS

1. $SaO_2 > 90\%$ assures an adequate arterial oxygen content. Avoid $FiO_2 > 0.6$ when possible.
2. PEEP improves oxygenation by recruiting lung volume. It may reduce cardiac output if the patient is inadequately volume-loaded.
3. Avoid overdistension of compliant lung units – volutrauma – by manipulating the respiratory rate, tidal volume, and I:E ratio. Ventilation strategies include permissive hypercapnia, PCV and IRV. Beware gas trapping.

FURTHER READING

Dreyfuss, D. and Saumon, G. (1992) Barotrauma is volutrauma, but which volume is the one responsible? *Intensive Care Med.*, 18 (3), 139–41.

Keogh, B. F. (1995) Modes of ventilation in adult respiratory distress syndrome. *Curr. Anaes. Crit. Care*, 6, 17–24.

Nightingale, P. (1994) Pressure-controlled ventilation – a true advance? *Clin. intensive care*, 5, 114–22.

NOTES

1.7 WEANING

J. GOLDSTONE MD FRCA
Senior Lecturer, Department of Anaesthesia
Consultant, Department of Intensive Care Medicine
Middlesex Hospital, UCL
London

CASE HISTORY

A 65-year-old man with a known history of COPD was admitted with acute respiratory failure requiring intubation and mechanical ventilation. A chest infection was treated with antibiotic therapy and resolved to the point where weaning was contemplated.

EXAMINATION FINDINGS

A trial of spontaneous breathing revealed a respiratory rate of 32/min, tidal volume of 305 ml, PaO_2 of 12.3 kPa (FiO_2 0.45), PEEP 5 cmH_2O. The patient became distressed after a further 15 minutes of spontaneous breathing and was reventilated. Three attempts at withdrawal of mechanical ventilation resulted in tachypnoea, distress, and reventilation, each after a short time.

WHAT FURTHER INVESTIGATIONS ARE REQUIRED AND WHAT STRATEGIES CAN BE ADOPTED

This patient immediately developed rapid shallow breathing during the initial assessment. This sign is common in patients who cannot sustain spontaneous breathing and[2] has been quantified and assessed prospectively by Yang and Tobin. The ratio of breathing frequency to tidal volume (measured in litres) is termed f/Vt. When f/Vt is less than 80, weaning is likely and contrasts to those who fail where f/Vt is > 105. In our patient, the f/Vt was 32 / 0.305 = 104. This suggested that weaning was unlikely.

A prospective test of weaning has two purposes; to pick out the patients who will succeed and to identify patients who will fail. f/Vt is sensitive (0.95) and as such will almost always identify patients who are able to breathe spontaneously. The specificity is lower (0.64), implying that some patients with a high f/Vt, indicating likely failure, will in fact breathe spontaneously.

Spontaneous breathing is dependent on three main elements; respiratory drive, the strength of the respiratory muscles, and the load applied to them during each breath. This is the framework used to investigate and diagnose patients who cannot be weaned or those who unexpectedly fail.

Drive. In pre-existing lung disease, respiratory drive is high, and in this patient it will have to be at an optimal level in order to wean successfully. Residual sedation and paralysing drugs will reduce the effective output to the respiratory muscles and may require time to be eliminated. Previous mechanical ventilation may result acutely in an artificially low $PaCO_2$. Cerebrospinal pH will then rise acutely and become alkaline. At this stage, if the patient is weaned, any rise in $PaCO_2$ will not be met with as great a rise in cerebrospinal $[H^+]$. Minute ventilation will thus rise to a lesser extent, an apparent decrease in central drive. Finally, excessive catabolism can result in a high $PaCO_2$ load which may not be eliminated in patients with a fixed ability to breathe.

Strength. The strength of the muscles is often reduced in the critically ill. In COPD, patients are wasted and the inspiratory muscles are reduced in size and weight. Further important reductions in the ability of the inspiratory muscles to generate pressure occurs if the muscle is excessively shortened or elongated. If the chest is overexpanded, the diaphragm is low and flat and cannot generate pressure optimally.

The strength of the inspiratory muscles can be measured by performing a maximal inspiratory manoeuvre against a closed airway, PI max. In the intubated patient PI max. is difficult to perform. An alternative technique to measure inspiratory pressures involves the measurement of inspiratory gasps. This requires the airway to be occluded for 24 seconds after previous preoxygenation. In this patient, maximum pressure generated during gasping was -30 cmH$_2$O. The normal range for PI max. is -40 to -120 cmH$_2$O. If, as in this case, the patient is only moderately weak and still cannot wean, there must be an additional cause for the weaning failure, for example, a high load applied to the respiratory muscles. Striated muscle can fail to develop force due to electrolyte disturbances. Hypophosphataemia, hypomagnesaemia, and hypocalcaemia can all depress striated muscle function and should be corrected. Hypercapnic acidosis has a depressive effect on muscle function and this has been demonstrated in man.

Although hypoxaemia alone may or may not depress muscle function, the combination of hypoxaemia and hypocapnia does, a situation which often occurs in patients failing to breathe spontaneously. Muscle function is also depressed by poor nutrition, catabolism, and atrophy. Nutrition should be instituted early. Completely inactive respiratory muscles decrease their maximum pressure generating ability by 50% after 11 days. Although activity has not been shown to alleviate this problem for the respiratory muscles, other muscle groups maintain bulk during low-grade continual exercise. The maintenance of some form of spontaneous breathing may therefore be beneficial.

Load. The work performed during breathing is increased during bronchospasm and this needs to be specifically excluded. The work performed inflating the lungs and overcoming airways resistance can be assessed by measuring dynamic compliance (Cdyn). During constant flow ventilation (as provided by most ITU ventilators) with no inspiratory pause, Cdyn = tidal volume/peak airway pressure – PEEP. Cdyn in this case was 36 ml/cmH$_2$O, and this level of load may well be unsustainable in moderately weak patients.

When patients fail to wean unexpectedly, underlying cardiac disease is often overlooked. Mechanical ventilation acts in some as a left ventricular assist, and left ventricular failure can be unmasked when the ventilator is abruptly withdrawn. Lemaire and co-workers measured haemodynamics during weaning and demonstrated that large increases in pulmonary artery wedge pressure occurred together with modest increases in cardiac index and heart rate. Successful weaning occurred in 9 of 15 patients after diuretic therapy succeeded in decreasing blood volume. Incipient heart failure should be excluded in patients who repeatedly fail weaning trials and this can be assessed invasively with the aid of a pulmonary artery catheter.

KEY POINTS

When investigating patients who are having difficulty weaning from artificial ventilatory support, consider possible problems under the headings, drive, strength, and load.

FURTHER READING

Lemaire, F., Teboul, J. L., Cinotti, L. *et al.* (1988) Acute left ventricular dysfunction during unsuccessful weaning from mechanical ventilation. *Anesthesiology*, **69** (2), 171–9.

Yang, K. L. and Tobin, M. J. (1991) A prospective study of indexes predicting the outcome of trials of weaning from mechanical ventilation. *N. Engl. J. Med.*, **324** (21), 1445–50.

Part 2 Trauma

2.1 MULTIPLE TRAUMA

D. R. GOLDHILL FRCA

Senior Lecturer; Honorary Consultant in Anaesthesia and Intensive Care
The London Hospital Medical College and the Royal London Hospital
London

CASE HISTORY

A 25-year-old female was found alone in her car, having collided with a tree. It took 1 hour to extricate her from the wreckage. During that time she was reportedly 'semi-conscious' but deteriorated in the ambulance. On arrival in the emergency room her BP was unrecordable, respiratory rate was 25/min, and she had a Glasgow coma score (GCS) of 5.

Initial emergency room resuscitation was according to advanced trauma life support (ATLS) protocols.

On admission to the ICU she was ventilated and unresponsive. She had been sedated and paralysed in the emergency room. An uncut 8 mm endotracheal tube (ETT), two large bore peripheral lines, and a supra pubic catheter were in place. She had three rib fractures, multiple pelvic ring fractures, and a compound fracture of the femur. The lateral cervical spine X-ray and CT scan of the head were reported as normal.

EXAMINATION FINDINGS

Pupils were equal and responsive; BP 90/60 mmHg; heart rate 125/min; core temperature 35°C.

INVESTIGATIONS

Biochemistry

Urea, electrolytes and glucose: normal
Hb   8.0g/dl.
Clotting screen: platelets 50×10^9
INR 1.7
APTT twice control

Arterial blood gases (FiO$_2$ 0.6)

PaO$_2$	10.0 kPa
PaCO$_2$	4.5 kPa
pH	7.2
BE	−12 mmol/l

DISCUSS MANAGEMENT AND TREATMENT

This patient has suffered major trauma with a predicted mortality (TRISS) of 70%. Multiple organ failure is likely. She is cold, tachycardic, relatively hypotensive, and anaemic. Her clotting is deranged, lung function abnormal, and she has a significant metabolic acidosis. Hypovolaemia is probable and aggressive resuscitation with warmed colloid, crystalloid, and blood should continue. Assessment of the adequacy of perfusion is imprecise and relies upon capillary return, palpation of peripheral pulses, BP, CVP, and urine output. Raised lactate levels and a base deficit are associated with poor perfusion. A pulmonary artery flotation catheter measuring pulmonary artery occlusion pressure (PAOP) and cardiac output is useful to guide therapy. Cardiac output must be restored and maintained. A normal or raised BP is desirable to maintain perfusion of the brain and other vital organs. Some intensivists aim for 'supranormal' goals of cardiac output, oxygen delivery, and oxygen consumption. Inotropic support is likely to be required to achieve desired levels of BP and cardiac output.

Her abnormal coagulation must be corrected with platelets and clotting factors. High fibrinogen degradation products (FDPs) raises the possibility of disseminated intravascular coagulation (DIC).

Prophylaxis against deep venous thrombosis should start as clotting returns to normal. Pelvic bleeding may be difficult to control, sometimes requiring intra-abdominal packs or other measures including arterial embolization or a military anti-shock trousers (MAST).

The pelvic and femoral fractures should be reduced and stabilized as early as the patient's condition allows. This minimizes bleeding and reduces the considerable risk of acute lung injury.

She has a degree of traumatic head injury on which hypoxic injury has been superimposed. There may be intra-abdominal haemorrhage, ileus, and lung contusion.

Mechanical ventilation must therefore be continued. Adequate sedation is necessary and paralysis may be indicated. The lateral cervical spine X-ray misses about 15% of fractures and the patient should be managed accordingly.

Renal failure is likely from myoglobinuria following entrapment, as well as hypoperfusion and hypoxia. Early restoration of renal perfusion and oxygenation is essential. A forced alkaline diuresis, if performed early, may be of benefit for myoglobinuria. Watch out for a compartment syndrome. A high urine output must be maintained if possible and low-dose dopamine and diuretics may help achieve this. Haemofiltration or dialysis may be necessary.

All wounds must be debrided and cleaned, blood cultures taken, and suitable antibiotic treatment continued. Selective decontamination of the digestive tract (SDD) is controversial but may prevent respiratory tract infections. Inadvertent one lung intubation is possible with an uncut tube which should be adjusted if necessary, securely fastened at the correct length, or cut to size.

Lines placed before admission to the ICU may be dirty and should be replaced. Injuries may be missed during the initial assessment or develop late. Be vigilant for haemo/pneumothorax, intracerebral or intra-abdominal pathology, or minor injuries such as broken fingers, lacerations, eye trauma, and glass in wounds. A female patient of this age may be pregnant. A car crash as described may be associated with alcohol, drugs, attempted suicide, or acute medical conditions such as epilepsy or a subarachnoid haemorrhage.

KEY POINTS

1. Continued resuscitation with colloid, crystalloid, and blood is usually necessary in the trauma patient. Even CVP and PAOP are poor indicators of the adequacy of resuscitation.
2. Hypotension, hypoxia, and a low cardiac output must be prevented.
3. Be vigilant for missed injuries.
4. Multiple organ failure is likely. The patient will probably get worse before she gets better!

FURTHER READING

Albou-Khalil, B., Scalcea, T. M., Trooskin, S. Z., Henry, S. M., et al. (1994) Haemodynamic responses to shock in young trauma patients. Need for invasive monitoring. Crit. Care Med., 22, 573–9.

Livingstone, D. H. (1993) Management of the surgical patient with multiple system organ failure. Am. J. Surg., 165 (2A), 8S–13S.

Riemer, B. L., Butterfield, S. L., Diamond, D. L., Young, J. C., et al. (1993) Acute mortality associated with injuries to the pelvic ring: The role of early patient mobilization and external fixation. J. Trauma, 35, 671–7.

NOTES

2.2 OXYGEN DELIVERY IN TRAUMA

D. WATSON FRCA
Consultant and Senior Lecturer in Anaesthesia and Intensive Care,
St. Bartholomew's and Homerton Hospitals
and

M. HAYES MD FRCA
Consultant Anaesthetist
Charing Cross Hospital
London

CASE HISTORY

A 30-year-old male fell from a third-floor window. On admission to hospital he was shocked but conscious. BP was 80/60 mmHg; pulse 120/min. X-ray of the pelvis revealed an acetabular fracture. Peritoneal lavage was positive for blood and laparotomy revealed a massive retroperitoneal haematoma. Prior to transfer to the angiography suite he had been transfused 27 units of packed red cells. Following successful arterial embolization, he was transferred intubated and ventilated to the ICU, where initial haemodynamic data were as follows:

INVESTIGATIONS

Mean arterial pressure	79 mmHg;
Core temperature	36°C;
Heart rate	110/min;
Urine output	100 ml in the preceding three hours.

Haemodynamic variables

Cardiac index	4 l/min/m^2
PAOP	7 mmHg
CVP	7 mmHg
Systemic vascular resistance index	1445 dynes.sec/cm^{-5}/m^2
Oxygen delivery index	474 ml/min/m^2
Oxygen consumption index	121 ml/min/m^2
Lactate	4.2 mmol/l
Hb	8.6 g/dl

DISCUSS MANAGEMENT AND TREATMENT

This young man has suffered life-threatening haemorrhage from trauma. He has required a massive blood transfusion and is at risk of sepsis and multiple organ failure, despite definitive surgical management. He is not yet resuscitated as evidenced by a tachycardia, low Hb, and raised lactate levels. (Normal lactate levels are below 2.0 mmol/l.)

The first priority must be to maintain an adequate airway and ventilation with continued cervical spine immobilization by a hard collar, sandbags, and tape across the forehead until the X-rays are reviewed by senior surgical staff and the possibility of cervical spine injury is excluded.

Volume expanders should be administered to an optimal left atrial pressure. This is taken as the PAOP at the plateau value for left ventricular stroke work index, whilst maintaining the Hb > 10 g/dl. The effects of transfusion on peripheral and central temperature, urine output, haemodynamics, oxygen transport, and lactate levels should be monitored. If the cardiac index were < 2.8 l/min/m^2 despite optimal fluid administration, some authorities recommend that dobutamine should be commenced (2.5–25 µg/kg/min) to maintain cardiac index in the range 2.8–3.5 l/min/m^2. (Incremental doses of dobutamine should cease if a tachycardia > 130 beats per minute, ECG evidence of myocardial ischaemia, or any tachydysrhythmias develop). At all times mean arterial pressure should be maintained greater than 80 mmHg even if this necessitates the infusion of noradrenaline (0.005–10 mcg/kg/min), whilst avoiding excessive vasoconstriction (systemic vascular resistance index > 1500 dynes.sec/ cm^{-5}/m^2).

Should these strategies succeed then sequential lactate levels and other markers for peripheral perfusion, e.g. peripheral temperature and urine output, will improve. If there is no improvement the possibility of non-vital tissue or continued haemorrhage should be explored.

KEY POINTS

1. It has been recognized for many years that survival following surgery is dependent on an adequate cardiac reserve. This finding has been repeatedly confirmed by Shoemaker et al. in critically-ill, postoperative patients. They also noted that survival was associated with higher levels of oxygen delivery (DO_2) and consumption (VO_2).

2. Pre-emptive therapy to increase oxygen transport before elective or emergency surgery to increase oxygen transport has been associated with improved survival. However, in a prospective randomized study involving heterogeneous groups of medical and surgical patients who were admitted postoperatively, or when complications prompted admission to an intensive care facility; if optimal filling was ensured and perfusion pressure well-maintained, dobutamine administration failed to influence oxygen consumption or lactate levels, nor did it improve clinical outcomes.

3. Recently, Gattinoni and his colleagues have carried out a large multicentre trial in three groups of critically-ill patients. In the control group the objective was to achieve normal haemodynamics (including a cardiac index of 2.5–3.5 l/min/m^2; in the second group a supranormal cardiac index (above 4.5 l/min/m^2) was the goal; and in the third group the intention was to maintain the mixed venous oxygen saturation at or above 70%.

This goal-orientated haemodynamic therapy did not influence morbidity or mortality; nor did it benefit patients in any of the predefined subgroups, including victims of trauma or postoperative patients. Inotrope therapy aimed at achieving anything other than normal haemodynamic values does not seem to be indicated in patients with established critical illness.

FURTHER READING

Boyd, O., Grounds, R. M., and Bennett, E. D. (1993) A randomized clinical trial of the effect of deliberate perioperative increase of oxygen delivery on mortality in high-risk surgical patients. *J.A.M.A.*, **270**, 2699–707.

Clowes, G. H. A. Jr. and Del Guericio, L. R. (1960) Circulatory response to trauma of surgical operations. *Metabolism*, **9**, 67–81.

Gattinoni, L., Brazzi, L., Pelosi, P., *et al.* (1995) A trial of goal-orientated haemodynamic therapy in critically-ill patients. *N. Engl. Med. J.*, **333**, 1025–32.

Hayes, M. A., Timmins, A. C., Yau, E. H. S., *et al.* (1994) Elevation of systemic oxygen delivery in the treatment of critically-ill patients. *N. Engl. Med. J.*, **330**, 1717–22.

Shoemaker, W. C., Montgomery, E. S., Kaplan, E., *et al.* (1973) Physiologic patterns in surviving and nonsurviving shock patients. *Arch. Surg.*, **106**, 630–6.

Shoemaker, W. C., Appel, P. L., Kram, H. B., *et al.* (1988) Prospective trial of supranormal values of survivors as therapeutic goals in high risk surgical patients. *Chest*, **94**, 1176–86.

NOTES

J. B. SALMON MRCP
Consultant Physician
Intensive Care Unit
The Royal Hospital Haslar
Gosport
Hampshire

CASE HISTORY

A 25-year-old man was admitted to A&E in a district general hospital following a road traffic accident in which he was the passenger. After initial assessment and colloid resuscitation in A&E he was conscious and haemodynamically stable. He was breathing with difficulty and complained of pain in the chest, and left leg. His injuries included numerous abrasions; compound fracture, left tibia; and closed fracture, left femur.

EXAMINATION FINDINGS

Peritoneal lavage was clear. Chest X-ray showed a small left-sided effusion and fractures to his left 1st–7th ribs. There was no flail segment.
Pelvis and cervical spine: no bony injury.

INVESTIGATIONS

Heart rate 120/min; BP 150/80 mmHg; CVP 12 mmHg; respiratory rate 35/min.

Electrolytes	normal
Hb	10.4 g/dl
Platelets	176×10^{-9}
WCC	12.6×10^{-9}
INR	1.7
CK	1500 iu/ml

Urine output 45ml in preceding hour
Blood +++ on dipstick testing

Arterial blood gases (FiO$_2$ 0.4)

PaO$_2$	12 kPa
PaCO$_2$	3.6 kPa
pH	7.38
BE	− 4.6 mmol/l

The ITU is full and the intention is to transfer him to another district general hospital 10 miles away where the fractures can be fixed and he can receive post-operative ITU care.

WHAT SHOULD BE DONE BEFORE THE TRANSFER AND HOW WOULD YOU CONDUCT IT?

This man is not fully resuscitated despite the normal urine output, BP, and CVP (he is tachycardic and has a compensated metabolic acidosis implying hypovolaemia). He is unstable and transfer is undesirable at this stage. He has at least four unresolved problems:

1. He needs further fluid resuscitation, preferably using dynamic volume challenges against the CVP or stroke volume.
2. The multiple fractures (especially the first rib) imply a high-speed injury. The pleural effusion probably represents a haemothorax and the combination raises the possibilities of damage to a major mediastinal vessel, cardiac or pulmonary contusion. He needs a chest CT scan urgently.
3. The blood on dipstick testing may represent myoglobin or haemoglobin. Although there was no blood on peritoneal lavage, it is still possible that he has intra-abdominal or retroperitoneal damage. This could be investigated by CT scanning at the same time as the chest CT. The low creatine kinase would suggest the danger of rhabdomyolysis is not great but he should be observed for evidence of compartment syndrome.
4. Ideally, the fractures of the left femur and tibia should be fixed before transfer.

Investigations should include baseline electrocardiogram (ECG) chest and abdominal CT (with contrast) and an echocardiogram if there is evidence of myocardial contusion. The pleural effusion on the left should be tapped and if bloody, drained. There are two transfers to be planned: (i) the initial intra-hospital transfer to the CT scanner, and (ii) a possible secondary transfer to another hospital later. There is a danger that he will deteriorate suddenly during the CT scan and it is essential that:

(i)   the scanner is ready to accept before he leaves the resuscitation area;
(ii) an experienced medical escort accompanies him;
(iii) adequate intravenous access, blood, colloids, and resuscitation equipment should be on hand.

Consideration should be given to intubating him electively before CT scanning as he will require intubation for operation later anyway and it may be better to intubate him in controlled circumstances now rather than risk an uncontrolled emergency intubation later. Monitoring during transfer and scanning should include ECG, continuous invasive arterial blood pressure, CVP, urine output, pulse oximetry, and end-tidal carbon dioxide ($EtCO_2$) measurement if intubated.

Whether or not he is transferred to another hospital depends on the results of the CT scan. Transfer should be considered immediately if the CT scan shows evidence of disruption of a major mediastinal vessel which cannot be managed locally. In this case, he should be transferred to a cardiothoracic centre: the district hospital 10 miles away may not be suitable. In these circumstances, he should be intubated and consideration given to controlling the BP during transfer with esmolol or sodium nitroprusside infusion. Clearly this is a hazardous undertaking in the acutely-injured patient and should be embarked on very cautiously, only after adequate volume resuscitation and discussion with the receiving unit.

Clotting disorders should be treated before departure and quantities of colloid and blood, including fresh frozen plasma (FFP) should be carried. However, in the event of a sudden vascular catastrophe during transit there may be little that can be done.

During transfer, monitoring should be continued as for the scanner. Sedation with paralysis is recommended if he is ventilated. An adequate transport ventilator should be used, capable of maintaining lung volumes over sustained periods. The emphasis should be on a smooth transit, avoiding sudden acceleration, deceleration, or fast cornering: a police escort is invaluable for this. The police should be briefed beforehand on what exactly is expected of them.

It is sensible to ensure that there is some means of communication between the ambulance and the receiving hospital. They must be given an estimated time of arrival (ETA). The exact destination of the patient on arrival (ICU or direct to X-ray or theatres) should be known and the door porters at the receiving end, briefed. Any alternative hospitals to which one could divert *en route* should be identified and their telephone numbers recorded. It is vital that all X-rays and scans accompany the patient.

If the CT scan is clear and he responds to resuscitation, the fractures should be fixed. If he still requires ventilatory support he could be transferred at this stage although a better option would be to move a more stable candidate who is on the ICU already. This often causes a dilemma. The advantage of transferring the most stable patient is that the risk of a deterioration *en route* is less. Conversely, if the stable patient deteriorates during transfer it is difficult to justify the move with relatives, who, anyway, may have developed a supportive relationship with the first ICU staff. There is also the risk of transferring multi-resistant organisms between units. The most stable patients are usually those who have been on the unit longest and have had the greatest opportunity to acquire resistant organisms.

TRANSFER CHECKLIST

1. **General.** Is this the most appropriate patient to transfer to the hospital in question? Is there anything that can be done to improve the patient's condition before transfer? Are the staff accompanying the patient sufficiently experienced? Is monitoring adequate and functioning?
2. **Oxygen and ventilation.** Prior to transportation, ventilate the patient on the transfer ventilator and ensure respiratory function remains stable. Most patients need to be transferred on 100% oxygen. Remember that at high inspired oxygen concentrations oximeters are slow to detect

pulmonary deterioration. Ensure enough oxygen is taken to ventilate the patient on 100% oxygen for at least twice the predicted duration of the transfer. Include 30 minutes for movement around the receiving hospital. Calculate the likely oxygen consumption of the transfer ventilator. Take an oxygen flowmeter and cylinder connection in case you have to hand-ventilate.

NB. Cylinder capacities (litres):

C	170 l
D	340 l
E	680 l
F/AF	1360 l
G	3400 l
J	6800 l

3. **Liaison.** Have you let the receiving hospital know you are on the way? Do they still have a bed? Is there a mobile telephone in the ambulance? Have you identified other hospitals *en route* to which you can divert if necessary? Has the situation been explained to the relatives?
4. **Drugs.** Have you got all the drugs you could conceivably need? Adrenaline and atropine are absolutely essential. Ensure the syringe and infusion pumps have sufficient battery life.
5. **Emergency equipment.** This should include an Ambu bag in working order, laryngoscopes, ET tubes, gum elastic bougies, monitors, a defibrillator and external pacemaker, chest drains, and portable suction.
6. **Notes.** Make sure you have notes, X-rays, blood/microbiology results, and any other documentation that may be relevant.

KEY POINTS

1. Ensure the patient is properly resuscitated before transfer.
2. Transfer the most stable patient if possible.
3. The commonest reasons for deterioration *en route* are inappropriate ventilation (wrong settings, wrong ventilator, disconnection), inadequate resuscitation, insufficient equipment/drugs, and inexperienced staff.
4. Preplan the journey and identify intermediate destinations.
5. Ensure you have some means of communication with base and receiving hospital.

FURTHER READING

Gilligan, J. E. (1990) Transport of the critically ill. In (ed. T. E. Oh) *Intensive care manual*, 3rd edn. Butterworth, Sydney.

Westaby, S. (1990) The injured heart. *Clin. Intensive Care*, 1(5), 210–19.

NOTES

N. McGuire FRCA
Consultant in Anaesthetics and Intensive Care
The Royal Hospital Haslar
Gosport
Hampshire

CASE HISTORY

A 23-year-old male was admitted to hospital following a fracture dislocation of the cervical spine, sustained when he dived into the shallow end of
a swimming pool. He had been on a backpacking holiday in the USA.
It was requested that he be repatriated to the UK, using an aeromedical
evacuation flight.

The aereomedical team was given the following information. There had
been a fracture dislocation of C3 on C4, with loss of all motor and sensory
function below this level. The injury had been stabilized using internal
fixation in the first 48 hours after the injury. Recovery had been complicated by bronchial plugging with secretions and a pulmonary infection
which was responding to physiotherapy and antimicrobial treatment. He
had been in hospital for 14 days.

CURRENT STATUS

Ventilatory assistance with CPAP of 5 cmH_2O and pressure support of 10
cmH_2O via a tracheostomy. FiO_2 0.48. Temperature 38.5°C; respiratory
rate 18/min. He was receiving naso-enteral tube feeding. Medications
included a third generation cephalosporin, heparin, and acetaminophen.

INVESTIGATIONS

Biochemistry

Sodium	128 mmol/l
Potassium	5.0 mmol/l
Chloride	109 mmol/l
Urea	5.1 mmol/l
Creatinine	70 μmol/l
Hb	9.4 g/dl
WCC	18.0×10^9/l
Platelets	100×10^9/l
INR	1.8

Arterial blood gases

PaO_2	9.3 kPa
$PaCO_2$	4.5 kPa
pH	7.32
BE	-6.4

IF YOU WERE THE PHYSICIAN RESPONSIBLE FOR THE FLIGHT, WHAT WOULD YOUR CONSIDERATIONS BE IN THIS CASE?

This young man has a number of problems including anaemia, hypoxia, hyponatraemia, and a metabolic acidosis. The INR is raised. He is also pyrexial despite treatment with antibiotics and chest physiotherapy, and has other markers of unresolved sepsis.

In this type of situation it is vitally important to obtain all clinically relevant information about the patient's condition. It is very easy to give into the releasing hospital's desire to facilitate the patient's departure. In their enthusiasm, some things may be glossed over unless the correct questions are asked.

If he has had an uncomplicated cervical spine injury, it is unlikely that he would be anaemic. Closer inspection of the patient's case notes reveals some intermittent lability of BP and pulse which was attributed to the cervical cord injury. If, however, one considers that the injury was followed by early surgery and almost immediate pulmonary sepsis it is clear that there may be associated problems. In fact sepsis has led to a raised INR and the patient is anticoagulated with heparin. A gastrointestinal bleed must therefore be high on the list of causes for the anaemia.

The correct course of events would be to perform upper gastrointestinal endoscopy to evaluate the gastrointestinal tract. Treat findings as appropriate. This may include H_2 antagonist therapy with continued feeding.

Adequately pursue and treat the sepsis. The original source of infection may not be the current one so a full sepsis screen plus line changes must be considered.

Whether to continue with the heparin is a difficult decision. There is a serious risk of venous thrombosis and pulmonary embolism in these patients but temporarily discontinuing therapy until the INR is normalizing may be a wise precaution.

The patient should not be moved until all these points have been addressed. There should also be a delay of between 48–72 hours following the last fall in haemoglobin so that continued bleeding may be discounted.

AEROMEDICAL CONSIDERATIONS

Most of the points relating to the transfer of the critically ill are equally applicable regardless of the mode of transportation. Full monitoring is obligatory and precautions to ensure that there are no inadvertent disconnections of the various attachments to the patient are fundamental. A pre-flight check to see if the patient tolerates the transport ventilator is well worthwhile. As part of the comprehensive range of equipment taken, an Ambu-bag in working order is an invaluable asset.

Oxygen. Unless you are lucky enough to have a dedicated aeromedical aircraft you will have to bring your own! The military usually take standard 1369 litre cylinders with all the potential connections which may be needed. The amount taken is calculated on a worst-case scenario for oxygen consumption. This includes amounts for unexpected hold-ups, diversions, etc. Remember that some ventilators driven by oxygen will have their own consumption as well as the patients minute volume to be taken into consideration. On long-haul flights the problem is the bulk of the cylinders and the means of restraining them.

Power. Electrical power supplies on aircraft are of various types. Establishing the voltage, number of outlets, need for adaptors, etc. is another issue which should be dealt with before setting off. Nickel cadmium batteries can usually be carried. Lead acid batteries are out.

General. The particular hazards associated with air travel depend to a degree on whether it is fixed wing (normal aircraft) or rotary wing (helicopter). Rotary wing aircraft are noisier and tend to be more prone to vibration. They are also less reliable as a stable platform. Despite these differences the problems associated with aeromedical evacuation may be largely summarized as follows:

Hazards

- Altitude
- Temperature
- Noise
- Vibration
- Visibility
- Unfamiliar environment

Altitude. On commercial flights cabin altitudes are usually kept between 6000–8000 feet. Military aeromedical flights may agree to maintain cabin altitude at sea level though there are penalties involved of significantly increased fuel costs and shorter ranges of travel. (Helicopters do not use pressurization as they fly at relatively low altitudes. However that is not to say that pressure changes may be ignored in all circumstances.)

Increasing altitude brings potential for hypoxia as the fall in the partial pressure of oxygen leads to an increase in volume of gas-filled cavities in the patient. A small pneumothorax will expand by 20% at 6000 feet. These should be drained to avoid acute respiratory decompensation.

Patients with pneumoperitoneum from recent abdominal surgery are also at risk. It is normally advised that 10 days be allowed between surgery and transport by aircraft not pressurized to sea level so that air can be re-absorbed. Air in the skull will also expand and fractures into the sinuses are therefore potential risk factors. Air in the endotracheal tube cuff is also susceptible to pressure changes. It is recommended that the cuff be gently filled with saline or that the pressure be monitored continuously during times of altitude change. Attending staff who cannot equalize pressure in the middle ear should not fly.

Temperature. During transfer to and from the aircraft there may be periods when the patient is exposed to extremes of temperature. In some rotary wing aircraft heating may be difficult and landing doors may be open for a time.

Noise and vibration are considerable problems, particularly in small, fixed-wing, and most rotary wing aircraft. These may interfere with communication, monitoring, and the function of supportive equipment. Vibration may prevent gravity-dependent intravenous fluid administration.

Visibility. In addition to sensory deprivation caused by noise, visibility may be limited. This will cause problems with direct patient observations and routine monitoring. More importantly, visual alarms may be obscured. This, added to the difficulties of monitoring auditory information may be disastrous.

Unfamiliar environment. This is perhaps the most important point. Individuals who have not been trained in aeromedical transfer are not equipped to give optimal care and may cope poorly with an emergency involving the patient. In a general emergency involving the aircraft, the untrained individual will be a liability both to themselves and other members of the team.

Guidelines for the transfer of patients are currently being drawn up by the Association of Anaesthetists.

KEY POINTS

1. Safe aeromedical evacuation of patients is based on accurate initial assessment and stabilization prior to any move. One can imagine the scenario of an acute gastrointestinal haemorrhage 2 hours out of Washington at 35 000 feet!
2. It is vitally important to obtain all clinically-relevant information before agreeing to take over responsibility for the patient. It is dangerously easy to give in to the releasing hospital's desire to expedite the patient's departure.
3. It is important to remember that diversion to the nearest hospital following an untoward incident cannot be relied on to salvage the situation.
4. Training is extremely important before embarking on aeromedical transfer.

FURTHER READING

Bristow, A., Baskett, P., Dalton, M., Ediss, P., Evans, I., *et al.* (1991) Medical helicopter systems: recommended minimal standards of patient management. *J. Roy. Soc. Med.*, **84**, 242–44.

Fromm, R. E., and Dellinger, R. P. (1992) Transport of critically ill patients. *J. Intensive Care Med.*, **7**, 223–33.

McGuire, N. M. and Garrard, C. S. (In press) Transport of the critically ill or unstable patient. In (ed. C. S. Garrard, P. Foex, and S. Westaby) *Principles and practice of critical care.* Blackwell Science, Oxford.

Morley, A. P. (1996) Prehospital monitoring of trauma patients: experience of a helicopter emergency medical service. *Br. J. Anaes.*, **76**, 726–30.

2.5 ELECTROCUTION AND BURNS

R. F. ARMSTRONG FRCA

R. F. ARMSTRONG FRCA
Consultant in Anaesthesia and Intensive Care
Middlesex Hospital
UCL
London

CASE HISTORY

A 25-year-old male electrician was admitted with burns sustained whilst maintaining an electrical plant in a factory. The history obtained from the firemen was of rescue from a smoke-filled room. He was unconscious at the time of rescue. There were signs of an electrical fire.

EXAMINATION FINDINGS

On admission he was covered in soot. There was a 40% skin surface burn, including face and neck. He was coughing up black sputum. Examination of the palate revealed soot particles. There was a deep burn on the right hand consistent with an electrical injury and a possible exit wound in the anterior surface of the left thigh. BP was 90/70 mmHg; pulse 120/min. GCS was 11.

Arterial blood gases (FiO$_2$ 0.6)

PaO$_2$	13.7 kPa
PaCO$_2$	3.5 kPa
pH	7.21
HCO$_3$	16 mmol/l
BE	-8
Saturation	100%
COHb	30%

DISCUSS MANAGEMENT AND TREATMENT

The airway. The history of receiving the injury in an enclosed space, burns in the danger zone around nose and lips, and carbonaceous sputum strongly suggests smoke inhalation. A high measured carboxyhaemoglobin (COHb) level supports the diagnosis though the level declines with time after the injury. (Note that pulse oximeters do not recognize COHb and overread. Blood gas analysers derive saturation from the oxygen tension and thus miss the presence of COHb).

Intubation of the trachea is indicated to protect against airway obstruction by oedema, especially as there is a reduced level of consciousness. In less clear-cut cases, serial nasendoscopy by an experienced operator can be used to monitor development of laryngeal or pharyngeal oedema. Although lethal hyperkalaemia following suxamethonium administration has not been reported during the first 24 hours after a burn, authorities do not recommend its use after 12 hours. Once intubated serial bronchial lavage can remove large amounts of soot and subsequently pieces of necrotic epithelium. Steroids are not used. Antibiotics are, when organisms are identified.

Poisoning. In view of the high carboxyhaemoglobin 100% oxygen should be given for 24 hours. Hyperbaric oxygen is recommended but may not be a practical option in the burned patient. The metabolic acidosis may be due to carbon monoxide poisoning, hypovolaemia, or may indicate cyanide poisoning. Cyanide levels take too long to measure so a clinical decision regarding antidotes has to be made. Experts disagree. Some suggest that normal supportive measures are sufficient treatment in cyanide poisoning. Others recommend antidotes, especially if there is a lactic acidosis. If antidotes are to be used, the safest available in the UK is sodium thiosulphate (50 ml 25% intravenously over 10 minutes). Nitrites produce methaemoglobin which mops up cyanide but reduces oxygen carriage. Dicobalt edetate produces inert complexes of cobalticyanide but in the absence of cyanide may cause cobalt poisoning.

Fluid management. In the UK, the Muir and Barclay plan divides up the first 24 hours into periods of 4,4,4,6,6 hours. In each period 0.5 ml/kg/% total body surface area (TBSA) burned is given as 4.5% albumin. The Parkland formula uses Hartmann's solution. 4 ml/kg/% TBSA burned is given over 24 hours; one half in the first 8 hours, the rest in the next 16. Both systems work well if fluid needs are constantly reassessed using standard objectives, i.e. pulse < 120/min; mean arterial pressure > 60 mmHg; $SpO_2 > 95\%$; urine output > 0.5 ml/kg; base deficit < 3.0mmol/l; mixed venous oxygen saturation $> 60\%$.

Electrocution. If the victim has fallen there may be associated fractures and blunt trauma including cervical spine injury. Neither the size of the entry and exit wounds nor the cutaneous burns are of help in deciding the extent of the injury. The course of the current through the body is unpredictable. There may be extensive internal injuries, i.e. gall bladder necrosis, bowel fistulae, or perforation. Cardiac muscle damage with ECG changes occurs in 30% of cases. Muscle damage is common with swelling causing compartment syndromes and nerve compression in arms and legs.

Tissue pressure measurements are helpful (a tissue pressure rising to within 30 mmHg of the diastolic pressure suggests dangerous swelling). Escharotomy in the ICU, fasciotomies in theatre, and the removal of dead and devitalized tissue is crucial. Surgical second and third looks may be necessary to identify dead tissue.

Creatine kinase (CK) measurement (> 10 000 iu/l) or positive dipstick urine tests for blood in the absence of red cells suggests rhabdomyolysis and indicates forced alkaline diuresis. Persistent metabolic acidosis or high lactate levels may indicate cryptic hypovolaemia or ischaemic tissue. Fluid needs in the electrically-injured patient may be much higher than calculated from surface area burned.

KEY POINTS

1. Repeated assessment of airway and fluid status is mandatory in the burned patient.
2. Poisoning may be a concurrent problem.
3. The electrocuted patient may have severe hidden injuries as well as blunt trauma. Repeated surgical exploration may be necessary.

FURTHER READING

Baud, F. J. *et al.* (1991) Elevated blood cyanide concentrations in victims of smoke inhalation. *N. Engl. J. Med.*, **325**, 1761–6.

Deitch, E. A. (1990) The management of burns. *N. Engl. J. Med.*, **323**, 1249–3.

McQueen, M. M. and Court-Brown, C. M. (1996) Compartment monitoring in tibial fractures. The pressure threshold for decompression. *J. Bone Joint Surg.*, **78**(B), 99–104.

Muller, M. J. and Herndon, D. M. (1994) The challenge of burns. *Lancet*, **343**, 216–20.

NOTES

2.6 HYPOTHERMIA

M. P. HAYWARD FRCS
Department of Cardiothoracic Surgery
Middlesex Hospital
UCL
London

CASE HISTORY

A 28-year-old woman was found, apparently dead, at 0700 hours on a park bench. The air temperature overnight was 2°C with continuous overnight rain. No discernible pulse could be felt but a passing policeman detected faint infrequent respiratory efforts. External cardiac massage was commenced and she was brought to the local A&E department. On admission she had no detectable cardiac output, was making no respiratory effort, and had fixed, dilated pupils. A low-reading rectal thermometer gave a core temperature below 28°C; ECG showed slow ventricular fibrillation. She was intubated and ventilated, and external cardiac massage was continued. There was no cardiac response to DC cardioversion or any standard resuscitation drugs.

INVESTIGATIONS

Biochemistry

Potassium	7.6 mmol/l
Sodium	139 mmol/l
Urea	6.9 mmol/l
Creatinine	108 μmol/l
WCC	20.0×10^9/l
Hb	11.0 g/dl
Platelets	256×10^9/l

Arterial blood gases (FiO$_2$ 1.0)

PaO$_2$	15 kPa
PaCO$_2$	8.9 kPa
BE	−28 mmol/l
pH	6.8

Cardiac massage and mechanical ventilation were continued for over an hour whilst unavailing attempts were made to rewarm the patient.

WHAT IS THE PROGNOSIS? DISCUSS MANAGEMENT AND TREATMENT

This woman's prognosis for complete recovery is very good (over 60%) if she is properly managed. Hypothermia, defined as a core temperature below 35°C, is not uncommon in patients attending UK casualty departments. It is implicated in 2000 deaths annually and is a complicating factor in 2.5–3.6% of all medical admissions during the winter months. Patient management is crucially dependent on an accurate assessment of core temperature, the presence of a circulation, and the underlying cause of the hypothermia.

Two main groups of hypothermic patients can be identified. The first comprises medically unwell patients who become hypothermic as a result of their medical condition. The majority are elderly. Mortality is up to 80%. The second group are previously healthy, young individuals or children who suffer accidental hypothermia (exposure, water immersion, snow burial) and in whom the recovery is excellent, even in cases of cardiac arrest for over 6 hours, core temperature as low as 15°C, and water immersion over an hour (provided ECM and ventilation is maintained).

Further management includes categorization of the patient into one of the above medical groups, an accurate assessment of the core temperature (CT), and the presence or absence of a circulation.

For all patients:

1. Reduce heat loss and further deterioration from the point of rescue.
2. Gentle handling – unnecessary manipulation can trigger lethal dysrrhythmias which may be refractory to treatment.
3. Warm, humidified oxygen should be given via an adequate airway.
4. Early I.V. access. All I.V. fluids should be warmed (to 37°C). Send full blood count; group and save serum, urea and electrolytes, glucose, amylase, calcium, magnesium, clotting and toxicology as a minimum. Blood gas and arterial BP monitoring are essential.
5. Establish the true core temperature (CT) and proceed as follows:

Mild hypothermia (CT 32 – 35°C). Use passive or active external warming methods – warmed insulation, external heated blankets, pads, radiant heaters, warm water immersion, or plumbed mattresses or garments. Consider reducing the problem of 'afterdrop' and intravascular volume depletion by actively rewarming the thorax alone.

Moderate hypothermia (CT 28 – 32°C). Use active internal warming methods. With a productive cardiac rhythm, use airway rewarming, gastric, peritoneal, bladder, and pleural lavage. Haemodialysis has been used successfully. In the face of an arrest rhythm, the elderly and medically-compromised patients will not usually survive even if thoroughly rewarmed. However, the younger 'accidental' group should be rewarmed using cardiopulmonary bypass in a cardiac unit (see below).

Severe hypothermia (CT 15 – 28°C) or cardiac arrest following rescue. Cardiopulmonary bypass should be used to rewarm all patients in the 'accidental' group if it is available. There is now enough evidence to support their immediate transfer by road or air to a cardiac centre (in the UK, no point is more than 2 hours from a cardiac centre by ambulance or helicopter). Rewarming should be stopped during transfer but cardiac massage should be continued at half the normal rate.

Of rewarmed patients, over 80% return to work or resume normal activities.

KEY POINTS

1. Commonly recognized complications of severe hypothermia include severe metabolic acidosis (secondary to prolonged hypoperfusion), hyperkalaemia, severe capillary leak syndromes, pancreatitis, pneumonia, and adult respiratory distress syndrome.
2. The metabolic disturbance may be gross: consideration should be given to early or elective haemofiltration even if urine is being produced.
3. Some complications may result from rewarming rather than the hypothermia itself. In particular, there is concern that using active internal rewarming in a patient with a very poor circulation may raise local metabolic activity above the ability of the circulation to support it. This may explain some of the case reports of gut ischaemia following hypothermia.

FURTHER READING

Baumgartner, F. J., Janusz, M. T., Jamieson, W. R. E. *et al.* (1992) Cardiopulmonary bypass for resuscitation of patients with accident hypothermia and cardiac arrest. *Can. J. Surg.*, **35**, 184–7.

Carneli, H. M. (1992) Accident hypothermia. *J. Paed.*, **120**, 671–9.

Jolly, B. T. and Ghezzi, K. T. (1992) Accident hypothermia. *Emerg. Med. Clin. North America*, **10**, 311–27.

NOTES

2.7 CARBON MONOXIDE POISONING

M. R. Hamilton-Farrell MRCP FRCA
Consultant Anaesthetist
Intensive Care Unit
Whipps Cross Hospital
London

CASE HISTORY

A 30-year-old woman was found unconscious at her home, by paramedics who had been called by the patient 10 minutes earlier. She rapidly regained consciousness after administration of oxygen by facemask, and by the time of admission to hospital had a GCS of 15. She appeared generally unwell and complained of a headache. She explained that she had not been well for 3 days before this incident. SpO_2 was 98%.

EXAMINATION FINDINGS

She appeared flat in affect, and her speech was monotonous. She was slow in her movements, although she could hold and drink a cup of tea. She had a pulse rate of 92/min and regular. Her short-term memory was impaired, but she was orientated in time and place. Her limb reflexes were uniformly brisk, but the plantar responses downgoing. She had blurring at the lateral margins of both optic discs. She was unable to walk heel-to-toe unaided, and Romberg's test was abnormal.

INVESTIGATIONS

Arterial blood gases (FiO$_2$ 0.6)

PaO_2	20.7 kPa
$PaCO_2$	3.8 kPa
pH	7.32
HCO_3	19.4 mmol/1
BE	-4.9 mmol/1
SaO_2	96%
COHb	32%

DISCUSS MANAGEMENT AND TREATMENT

Accidental carbon monoxide (CO) poisoning from domestic heating systems is often preceded by a period of ill-health, due to increasing exposure to leaking boiler exhaust gas. Flu-like symptoms may be wrongly dismissed as insignificant. Cherry-red skin colour is unusual. Circumstantial evidence of a source of carbon monoxide, combined with a carboxyhaemoglobin (COHb) level > 10% (15% in smokers) makes the diagnosis likely.

CO is not distinguished from oxygen by a pulse oximeter, or by the calculated SaO_2 given in blood gas results. Only a co-oximeter will reveal COHb levels. A metabolic acidosis is common. The severity of poisoning is not, however, reflected by the COHb level, the value of which depends mostly on the latest exposure, the delay before the sample is taken, and the interim administration of oxygen.

A history of loss of consciousness, however brief, is the most serious adverse prognostic factor. It may represent an ischaemia-reperfusion injury to the central nervous system which, combined with CO delivered via haemoglobin and plasma, is thought to lead to long-term pathology and late sequelae. Other bad prognostic factors include neurological abnormalities on admission (such as those illustrated in the case), myocardial ischaemia or arrhythmias, and pregnancy. Haemoglobin F has a higher affinity for CO than haemoglobin A, and fetal abnormalities may result. Headache alone is not significant, representing the cerebral oedema which is almost universal.

Late sequelae may arise in the days and weeks after apparent immediate recovery from CO poisoning. These are very difficult to treat, and can be devastating. Memory loss and coordination disturbances are most common; but psychiatric problems, parkinsonism, and epilepsy may result. The incidence of late sequelae is up to 40% over 3 years. It is principally to prevent this that hyperbaric oxygen (HBO) is indicated.

In every diagnosed case, 100% oxygen (via a cushion-rimmed mask with reservoir bag), should be given for 6–12 hours. Unconscious patients should always be intubated and artificially ventilated, at least to ensure adequate oxygen administration. General resuscitative measures are also essential. Discussion of patients with a hyperbaric oxygen facility is based on any one of the following:

- loss of consciousness at any stage
- neurological symptoms or signs other than a simple headache
- myocardial ischaemia or arrhythmias
- pregnancy
- COHb > 25%

The benefits and risks of patient transfer can then be considered.

Parasuicidal patients are generally returned to the referring hospital after HBO treatment, for psychiatric attention. Accidental victims may return home directly after HBO, which will also shorten the total duration of admission to hospital.

KEY POINTS

1. The diagnosis of accidental carbon monoxide poisoning is often missed in the first instance.
2. COHb levels do not reflect the severity of poisoning, or its prognosis.
3. Hyperbaric oxygen is indicated in severe cases, to reduce the risk of late sequelae.

FURTHER READING

Barret, L., Danel, V., and Faure, J. (1985) Carbon monoxide poisoning, a diagnosis frequently overlooked. *Clin. Toxicol.*, **23**, 309.

Brown, S. D. and Piantadosi, C. A. (1989) Reversal of carbon monoxide-cytochrome C oxidase binding by hyperbaric oxygen *in vivo*. *Adv. Exp. Biol. Med.*, **248**, 747–54.

Thom, S. R., Taber, R. L., Mendigruen, I. I., Clark, J. M., Hardy, K. R. and Fisher, A. B. (1995) Delayed neuropsychologic sequelae after carbon monoxide poisoning. Prevention by hyperbaric oxygen. *Ann. Emerg. Med.*, **4**, 474–80.

NOTES

2.8 THE HIGH-RISK SURGICAL CASE

O. BOYD MRCP FRCA
St George's Hospital
London

CASE HISTORY

A 75-year-old female presented to the surgical team with a 12-hour history of abdominal pain. She took regular NSAIDS for osteoarthritis. One year previously she was admitted to the same hospital with a myocardial infarction, since when she had taken regular frusemide and enalapril for shortness of breath. She lived in a bungalow with social services support.

EXAMINATION FINDINGS

Pulse rate 120/min; BP 100/50 mmHg; temperature 38°C; respiratory rate 25/min with shallow breaths and decreased air entry at the bases. Auscultation revealed a gallop rhythm and the abdomen was tense and silent.

INVESTIGATIONS

Biochemistry

Hb	10.0 g/dl
WCC	$15.3 \times 10^9/l$
Sodium	136 mmol/l
Potassium	4.8 mmol/l
Chloride	100 mmol/l
Urea	15.0 mmol/l
Creatinine	170 μmol/l
Bicarbonate	20 mmol/l

ECG: left bundle branch block, sinus rhythm
Chest X-ray: enlarged heart with gas under the diaphragm

THE SURGICAL TEAM WISH TO TAKE THE PATIENT TO THEATRE IMMEDIATELY WITH A DIAGNOSIS OF PERFORATED VISCUS, PROBABLY DUODENAL ULCER. THE PATIENT HAS SIGNED A CONSENT FORM. DISCUSS ADDITIONAL PREOPERATIVE MANAGEMENT

The patient has peritonitis requiring an operation. Perioperative management is controversial. She has congestive cardiac failure, renal impairment which may be acute or long standing, anaemia, and osteoarthritis. There is a metabolic acidosis possibly due to renal impairment or more probably representing a lactic acidosis.

Elderly patients with multiple pathology commonly present for emergency operations, and have a high postoperative mortality rate. This is usually the result of slow postoperative degeneration of organ function. The prognosis can be improved by optimizing cardiovascular function, by increasing oxygen delivery ($SaO_2 \times Hb \times Cl \times 0.134$) towards a target of 600 ml/min/m^2.

MANAGEMENT

A delay in surgery of 1–2 hours is acceptable as it will improve her prognosis. The patient is admitted to intensive care.

A 14 G peripheral line is sited, bloods are drawn for cross-match, clotting screen, lactate, and blood cultures. An arterial line, urinary catheter, and pulmonary artery flotation catheter are sited.

The blood tests reveal normal clotting times; lactate 2.1 mmol/l; pH 7.32; PaO_2 8.9 kPa; $PaCO_2$ 4.0 kPa; SaO_2 90%. Invasive measurements show CVP +2 mmHg; PAOP 9 mmHg; cardiac index (CI) 2.1 l/min; mean arterial pressure 68 mmHg; oxygen delivery is 253 ml/min/m^2. This suggests a lactic acidosis with intravascular volume depletion, low cardiac output, and pulmonary shunting. Inspired oxygen is increased. Intravascular volume is expanded by fluid challenges. Colloid is used, but in this anaemic patient, blood is given when available. The PAOP is targeted to 13–15 mmHg and CI increases to 2.5 l/min/m^2. In this patient, with a history of cardiac failure, further challenges are given. At a PAOP of 18, CI peaks at 2.7 l/min/m^2 and heart rate falls to 100/min. Oxygen delivery is 306 ml/min/m^2. Both Hb and cardiac output are low. Blood is therefore transfused and cardiac output increased with inotropes. Dopexamine, an 'inodilator', is chosen with a limit of an increase in heart rate of 20%. At 1.5 mcg/kg/min, CI is 3.6 l/min/m^2 and heart rate is 120/min. Oxygen delivery is 493 ml/min/m^2. This is the maximum achieved without causing a tachycardia. The patient can now proceed to operation.

1. Elderly patients with coexisting disease have a high perioperative mortality of up to 30%, usually from a slow degeneration of organ function.
2. Mortality can be reduced if perioperative care is targeted towards increasing tissue perfusion. A suitable target is an oxygen delivery of greater than 600 ml/min/m^2, as long as tachycardia is avoided.

FURTHER READING

Boyd, O., Grounds, R. M., and Bennett, E. D. (1993) A randomized clinical trial of the effect of deliberate perioperative increase of oxygen delivery on mortality in high-risk surgical patients. *JAMA.*, 270, 2699–707.

Scalea, T. M., Simon, H. M., Duncan, A. O., Atweh, N. A., Sclafani, S. J. A., Phillips, T. F., *et al.* (1990) Geriatric blunt trauma: Improved survival with early invasive monitoring. *J. Trauma*, 30, 129–36.

Shoemaker, W. C., Appel, P. L., Kram, H. B., Waxman, K., and Lee, T. S. (1988) Prospective trial of supranormal values of survivors as therapeutic goals in high-risk surgical patients. *Chest*, 94, 1176–86.

NOTES

Part 3 Cardiovascular

3.1 HYPOVOLAEMIA

A. WEBB MD MRCP
Clinical Director of Intensive Care
Middlesex Hospital
UCL
London

CASE HISTORY

A 32-year-old female patient was admitted to the ICU from the A&E department. She had presented after collapsing with left loin pain. She had a past history of recurrent urinary tract infections.

EXAMINATION FINDINGS

Pyrexia 38.0°C; pulse 130/min; sinus rhythm respiratory rate 24/min; BP 70/40 mmHg. Jugular venous pulse not visible. Heart sounds normal with no added sounds. Chest normal. Abdomen tender to palpitation in the left loin. Central nervous system normal other than mild drowsiness.

INVESTIGATIONS

Biochemistry		Arterial blood gases (FiO$_2$ 0.4)	
Sodium	143 mmol/l	PaO$_2$	14.3 kPa
Potassium	3.7 mmol/l	PaCO$_2$	3.1 kPa
Urea	9.2 mmol/l	pH	7.24
Creatinine	75 μmol/l		

WHAT IS THE MOST LIKELY CAUSE OF THE HYPOTENSION?

The patient was clearly hypovolaemic (hypotension, tachycardia, high haemoglobin, and high urea with normal creatinine). The history of recurrent urinary tract infection and the pyrexia, high white count, left loin pain, and tenderness suggest that a urinary infection is the main underlying diagnosis. Hypovolaemia may be due to polyuria associated with a urinary tract infection and peripheral vasodilatation associated with the pyrexia could have contributed to the hypotension. However, in this case, the presence of metabolic acidosis and thrombocytopenia suggest systemic septicaemia. Hypovolaemia in this situation is probably due to capillary leak and hypotension is probably due in part to hypovolaemia and in part to failure of compensatory peripheral vasoconstriction.

WHAT SHOULD THE INITIAL CARDIOVASCULAR MANAGEMENT BE?

Since there is a clear hypovolaemic component to this patient's cardiovascular disturbance, immediate fluid resuscitation is required. The choice of fluid for resuscitation should be a colloid to allow rapid intravascular volume correction. Given that capillary leak is likely, a colloid fluid containing larger molecules (a hydroxyethyl starch) should be chosen ideally. Gelatins and albumin both have short lives in the face of capillary leak and provide little advantage over crystalloid. It would be most appropriate to control plasma volume expansion by intermittent rapid infusions of 200 ml of colloid, observing the response of measured haemodynamic variables to each infusion (fluid challenge). The usual variables chosen would be CVP or the combination of stroke volume and pulmonary artery occlusion pressure.

In this particular case, however, none of these are being monitored. With such clear hypovolaemia, it would be reasonable to give up to two 200 ml infusions, observing clinical response initially. Failure of the BP to improve or heart rate to fall requires that further, invasive haemodynamic monitoring is instituted. Insertion of a central venous catheter becomes mandatory and insertion of a pulmonary artery catheter ideal. The correct interpretation of haemodynamic data allow rapid plasma volume expansion without the dangers of excessive fluid transfusion.

With CVP measurements it is best to observe changes in response to the rapid colloid infusion rather than aim for a specific CVP. We know nothing of the peripheral venous tone and myocardial compliance in the individual and therefore do not know the correct CVP to aim for. A sustained rise of CVP of 3 mmHg or more in response to a 200 ml fluid challenge suggests that the venous circulation is full and further fluid resuscitation may not be appropriate.

The pulmonary artery catheter allows fluid challenges to be controlled according to the response of stroke volume and pulmonary artery occlusion pressure. The comments made for the CVP above apply to interpretation of the pulmonary artery occlusion pressure. The optimum stroke volume that can be achieved in response to a fluid challenge is the maximum. Therefore, any increase in stroke volume in response to a fluid challenge should be a prompt to repeat the fluid challenge. No increase in stroke volume and a 3 mmHg or more rise in pulmonary artery occlusion pressure suggests the circulation is adequately filled.

IF HYPOTENSION PERSISTS AFTER INITIAL RESUSCITATION, WHAT FURTHER CARDIOVASCULAR MANAGEMENT WILL BE REQUIRED?

Persistent hypotension after adequate fluid resuscitation will require inotropic or vasopressor support. Optimum fluid resuscitation, as discussed above, achieved maximum stroke volume. If, however, this maximum stroke volume was less than normal (less than 60–70 ml) the possibility exists to increase it further with an inotrope. If stroke volume is normal and hypotension persists, it would be more appropriate to constrict the peripheral circulation with a vasopressor. Adrenaline will provide inotropic support whilst noradrenaline is predominantly a vasopressor. The drugs should be titrated against observed effect – aiming for a normal stroke volume with adrenaline and aiming for an adequate BP with noradrenaline. Defining an adequate BP presents a difficult problem, since we do not really know what is adequate for the individual. While normal would clearly be adequate, excessive doses of vasopressor required to achieve normal may compromise blood flow to some organs. A minimum mean arterial pressure of 60 mmHg would be a reasonable starting point with further increments in dose if the patient was previously hypertensive or if there are clinical benefits witnessed (such as correction of oliguria).

FURTHER READING

Haupt, M. T. and Rackow, E. C. (1982) Colloid osmotic pressure and fluid resuscitation with hetastarch, albumin, and saline solutions. *Crit. Care Med.*, 10, 159.

Meadows, D., Edwards, J. D., Wilkins, R. G., *et al.* (1988) Reversal of intractable septic shock with norepinephrine therapy. *Crit. Care Med.*, 16, 663.

Sturm, J. A. and Wisner, D. H. (1985) Fluid resuscitation of hypovolaemia. *Intensive Care Med.*, 11, 227.

NOTES

3.2 MYOCARDIAL INFARCTION

M. SINGER MD MRCP
Senior Lecturer in Intensive Care Medicine
Bloomsbury Institute of Intensive Care Medicine
UCL Medical School
London

CASE HISTORY

A 55-year-old man is admitted with a 1-hour history of crushing central chest pain and breathlessness. There is a past history of duodenal ulcer surgery 5 years previously and recent onset anginal symptoms. On arrival he is drowsy, tachypnoeic (30/min), tachycardic (120/min), and hypotensive (70/45 mmHg). Auscultation reveals widespread end-inspiratory crackles and a gallop rhythm.

INVESTIGATIONS

Biochemistry		Arterial blood gases (FiO$_2$ 0.6)	
Potassium	3.5 mmol/l	PaO$_2$	8.4 kPa
Sodium	140 mmol/l	PaCO$_2$	5.2 kPa
Urea	5.3 mmol/l	HCO$_3$	12 mmols/l
Glucose	8.2 mmols/l	BE	−10
Creatine kinase	400 IU/l	pH	7.27

ECG: leads V1-V4 show q waves, ST elevation, T wave inversion.
CXR: cardiomegaly, engorged pulmonary vessels, Kerley B lines, upper lobe diversion.

DISCUSS MANAGEMENT AND TREATMENT

A diagnosis of a large anteroseptal myocardial infarction (MI) can be made from the history and ECG findings. The CPK level is elevated but, being taken shortly after chest pain onset, can be expected to rise further. The hypotension and hypoperfusion (drowsiness, metabolic acidosis) are suggestive of cardiogenic shock. The patient is tiring (inappropriate hypercapnia for severe metabolic acidosis).

Priorities

1. ABC:

   (a) High flow, high concentration oxygen. As the patient is tiring, early institution of CPAP or mechanical ventilation with PEEP would be beneficial to reduce the work of breathing, venous return, and left ventricular afterload;

   (b) Large bore cannulation of good peripheral vein;

   (c) 'Empiric' institution of inotropes until adequate BP restored (i.e. mean BP > 60 mmHg) – e.g. adrenaline (2 mg diluted in 50 ml) initially given as small boluses (0.5–1 ml) followed by continuous infusion. If BP 'overshoots' wait 1–2 minutes for effect to wear off. Dobutamine can be used as an alternative (e.g. 5 μg/kg/min infusion doubling every 5 minutes until satisfactory BP achieved) though caution should be applied as this drug may cause vasodilatation and further hypotension.

2. Prompt central venous cannulation with 7.5 Fr sheath for pulmonary artery catheter (PAC) – should be inserted by experienced operator because of thrombolysis to follow, ideally in internal jugular vein.

3. Thrombolytic therapy – rTPA followed by heparin is preferable in this situation as there may be an early need for further invasive interventions (q.v.). The potential for peptic bleeding is low and the risks are outweighed by the potential benefits.

4. Contact cardiologist for:

   (a) echocardiogram to confirm presence (if any) of valve damage;

   (b) possibility of early angioplasty (depends on local policy);

   (c) consideration of early insertion of intra-aortic balloon pump.

5. Insertion of PAC and titration of treatment (inotropes ± dilators ± fluid) according to data obtained. Common findings would be a low cardiac output (< 3.5 l/min), an elevated PAOP (> 20 mmHg), an elevated systemic vascular resistance (> 1500 dyn.sec.cm^{-5}), and a low mixed venous oxygen saturation (SvO$_2$ – normal 70–75%). Target values for therapy: (i) SvO$_2$ ≥ 60% implying satisfactory oxygen delivery to meet demand; (ii) mean BP of 60–65 mmHg (may need to be higher in chronically hypertensive patient where oliguria or ST segment elevation remains). A PAOP of 15–20 mmHg is usually satisfactory but, rather than aiming for a set value, this should be titrated against

100–200 ml fluid challenges or varying vasodilator infusions to obtain optimal stroke volume (NB. small monitored fluid challenges will not produce 'crashing' pulmonary oedema). The PAOP may need to be higher to produce optimal stroke volume in a non-compliant ventricle. The patient often has coexisting hypovolaemia (sweating, vomiting, mouth breathing, frusemide given in Casualty) and this should be considered early as the cause of the hypotension and oliguria. A fall in BP following a small dose of vasodilator is also suggestive of hypovolaemia. Diuretics are usually not needed in acute management unless patient is on long-term diuretics.

6. After 24–48 hours, when the inotrope requirement has reduced, cautious addition of a short-acting ACE inhibitor such as captopril may be tried, initially at low dose, and then escalating to full dosage while any intravenous vasodilator infusion is weaned. Diuretics may be needed after the patient has been loaded with the ACE inhibitor.

7. Wean slowly from ventilator. Will probably need CPAP after extubation.

FURTHER READING

Bussman, W. and Schupp, D. (1978) Effect of sublingual nitroglycerin in emergency treatment of severe pulmonary oedema. *Am. J. Cardiol.*, **41**, 931–6.

Chatterjee, K., Swan, H. J. C., Kaushik, V. S., Jobin, G., Magnusson, P., and Forrester, J. S. (1976) Effects of vasodilator therapy for severe pump failure in acute myocardial infarction on short-term and late prognosis. *Circulation*, **53**, 797–802.

Dikshit, K., Vyden, J. K., Forrester, J. S., Chatterjee, K., Prakash, R., and Swan, H. J. C. (1973) Renal and extrarenal haemodynamic effects of furosemide in congestive heart failure after acute myocardial infarction. *N. Engl. J. Med.*, **288**, 1087–90.

Johnson, S. A., Scanlon, P. J., Loeb, H. S., Moran, J. M., Pifarre, R., and Gunnar, R. M. (1977) Treatment of cardiogenic shock in myocardial infarction by intra-aortic balloon counterpulsation and surgery. *Am. J. Med.*, **62**, 687–92.

Lee, L., Bates, E. R., Pitt, B., Walton, J. A., Laufer, N., and O'Neill, W. W. (1988) Percutaneous transluminal coronary angioplasty improves survival in acute myocardial infarction complicated by cardiogenic shock. *Circulation*, **78**, 1345–51.

Nelson, G. I. C., Ahuja, R. C., Silke, B., Hussain, M., and Taylor, S. H. (1983) Haemodynamic advantages of isosorbide dinitrate over frusemide in acute heart failure following myocardial infarction. *Lancet*, i, 730–2.

Singer, M. (1983) The management of acute heart failure: an iconoclastic view. *Care Crit. III*, **9**, 11–16.

NOTES

3.3 AORTIC DISSECTIION

M. P. HAYWARD FRCS
Department of Cardiothoracic Surgery
Middlesex Hospital
UCL
London

CASE HISTORY

A 59-year-old man was admitted to ITU from the A&E department. At the time of admission to A&E, his history was of collapse at home with sudden, severe chest pain radiating to his back, neck, and jaw. He was overweight and had smoked 20 cigarettes daily for 40 years. He gave a history of hypertension for 10 years. He was cool, sweaty, and in pain.

EXAMINATION FINDINGS

Pulse 110/min; BP 150/90 mmHg (both arms); soft non-tender abdomen. No neurological abnormalities except for weakness and tingling in the left arm. An initial ECG (during pain) showed non-specific ST - T changes in the lateral leads only.

Whilst in A&E his pain became much worse. He became tachypnoeic and increasingly distressed. A further ECG showed hyperacute ST - T changes in the anterior chest leads.

He was treated with high concentration oxygen and small doses of intra-venous diamorphine. A central venous cannula was placed in the right internal jugular vein and an arterial cannula in the right radial artery. CVP was 0 mmHg, BP was now 170/105 mmHg. Catheterization revealed a small volume of concentrated urine.

INVESTIGATIONS

Urea and electrolytes, full blood count, and clotting were normal. Chest X-ray showed a widened upper mediastinum and left pleural effusion.

DISCUSS MANAGEMENT AND TREATMENT

Although this man has obvious risk factors for coronary artery disease, there are several atypical features. The initial ECG taken during pain showed no significant acute changes. The interscapular pain and the widened upper mediastinum should raise the possibility of aortic dissection. Interscapular pain occurs in dissections both of the ascending and descending aorta, although it is more common in the latter. Pain radiating to the neck and jaw is almost specific for ascending aortic involvement. Unequal pulses are held to be a feature of dissection but are present in only approximately one-third, the femoral pulse being affected twice as frequently as the radial or subclavian. Other features suggesting dissection include aortic incompetence, acute neurological disturbances, and evidence of limb or organ ischaemia.

In this case the patient's initial pain stemmed from an acute dissection in the ascending aorta. The original ECG changes were longstanding whilst the subsequent deterioration and acute ECG changes were due to the dissection extending to involve the coronary arteries.

Any patient suspected of having aortic dissection should be admitted to an ITU. Pain should be relieved with incremental doses of intravenous diamorphine, oxygen should be given and blood (10 units) cross-matched. The arterial BP should be lowered immediately, aiming for a systolic BP < 120 mmHg and a mean arterial pressure < 80–90 mmHg (less if urine production can be maintained). The aim is not only to reduce BP (and hence wall stress) but also continued shearing forces. Intravenous sodium nitroprusside is the most convenient drug but intravenous beta blockers have a place, esmolol being the best choice.

An arterial cannula should be placed, not only to allow close BP monitoring, but also to allow sequential blood gas measurement seeking evidence of circulatory insufficiency.

Upon stabilization, preparations should be made for immediate transoesophageal echocardiogram, CT scan, or angiography.

Dissection usually originates in one of two locations – either in the ascending aorta within a few centimetres of the aortic valve or in the descending aorta just beyond the left subclavian artery. The Stanford classification is: Type A, dissections that involve the ascending aorta with varying degrees of distal extent; and Type B, dissections in which the ascending aorta is spared.

Transoesophageal echocardiography (TOE). This is the investigation of choice, particularly in tertiary referral centres. It can establish a prompt bedside diagnosis, visualize the intimal flap, the extent and type of dissection, entry tear, aortic valve, and coronary ostia. It may also be the definitive or only possible investigation in severely-ill patients.

Contrast enhanced CT. The investigation of choice if TOE is not available. Allows a quick and accurate assessment of the true and false lumina and the intimal flap between the two.

Angiography. Supplies an accurate diagnosis in 95–99% of cases. Can locate the intimal tear and extent of the false lumen, assess blood flow in the major vessels, and quantify aortic incompetence when present. Newer imaging modalities have superseded angiography in recent years.

Magnetic resonance imaging (MRI). Provides an accurate assessment of the situation in multiple planes and of the cardiac chambers and valves. It is impractical in the unstable patient but useful for diagnosing and following chronic dissection, particularly type B.

Definitive treatment. Surgical repair is the treatment of choice for all dissections involving the ascending aorta. One month survival is only 8% in the untreated patient. Medical therapy is the primary treatment for descending thoracic dissections, survival being 75% whether medical or surgical treatment is employed. Surgery is reserved for those who suffer the complications of compromised blood supply to vital organs or a limb or persistent pain. Severe neurological signs (dense stroke or paraplegia) are not an indication for surgery.

Principles of surgical treatment. The treatment is palliative, its purpose to prevent rupture, re-establish blood flow in ischaemic areas, and to protect the coronary arteries and aortic valve. Excision of the portion of aorta involved in the initial tear, reconstitution of the wall of the dissected aorta, and insertion of a prosthetic interposition graft is achieved with cardiopulmonary bypass. Involvement of the aortic valve requires either its resuspension or replacement with a valved conduit and re-implantation of the coronary ostia. Deep hypothermic circulatory arrest is used to carry out more extensive distal surgery of the aortic arch.

FURTHER READING

Erbe, R. (1993) Role of transoesophageal echocardiography in dissection of the aorta and evaluation of degenerative aortic disease. *Cardiol. Clin.*, **11** (3), 461–73.

Kirklin, J. W. and Barratt-Boyes, B. G. (1993) *Cardiac surgery*, 2nd edn. Churchill Livingstone, New York.

Leonard, J. C. and Hasleton, P. S. (1979) Dissecting aortic aneurysms: a clinico-pathological study. I. Clinical and gross pathological findings. *Quart. J. Med.*, **189**, 55–63.

Svensson, L. G., Crawford, E. S., Hess, K. R., Loselli, J. S., and Sagi, H. J. (1990) Dissection of the aorta and dissecting aortic aneurysms: Improving early and long-term surgical results. *Circulation*, **82** (IV), 24–38.

NOTES

3.4 RIGHT VENTRICULAR INFARCTION

H MONTGOMERY MRCP
Honorary Senior Registrar in Cardiology/ICU
Intensive Care Unit
Middlesex Hospital
UCL
London

CASE HISTORY

A 46-year-old man with a past history of hypertension presents with a 4-hour history of typical cardiac chest pain. The ECG shows ST elevation in the inferior leads consistent with an acute myocardial infarction, and he is treated with streptokinase at once. BP at presentation is 170/110 mmHg. Over the subsequent 30 hours, his pain continues despite treatment with intravenous nitrates and opioids. BP then slowly falls reaching 90/60 mmHg at 48 hours, a mounting sinus tachycardia develops, and he complains of breathlessness. A urinary catheter is inserted, upon which urine flow is found to be negligible.

EXAMINATION FINDINGS

The patient is cool peripherally. The pulse character is of sharp upstroke but low volume. The jugular venous pressure is elevated to the earlobes. There is an audible third heart sound. The apex beat is undisplaced and dynamic. The patient is tachypnoeic, pink on 28% inspired oxygen, and the lungs are clear. BP on arrival has fallen to 50/30 mmHg.

INVESTIGATIONS

Chest X-ray is unremarkable. The ECG shows an evolving inferior myocardial infarction.

Arterial blood gases (FiO$_2$ 0.28)

pH	6.96
PaCO$_2$	2.8 kPa
PaO$_2$	20.3 kPa
HCO$_3$	11 mmol/l

The patient is transferred to your care.

WHAT IS THE LIKELY DIAGNOSIS?

The patient has suffered a right ventricular myocardial infarction. The right ventricle (RV) has important function quite independent of that of the left ventricle (LV). RV ischaemic damage thus significantly worsens prognosis in any case of ischaemic cardiac failure, post-infarction ventricular septal defect, or LV infarction.

In cases of inferior myocardial infarction (MI), RV infarction increases mortality and morbidity five to sevenfold. RV infarction is more likely in those with known respiratory disease or sustained pre-existing RV burden. The left anterior descending artery supplies the RV infundibulum, the upper septum, and anterior 2–3 cm of RV which adjoins the septum. However, the bulk of the RV tends to be supplied by the right coronary artery (RCA), and the more proximal the RCA occlusion, the more likely severe RV damage becomes.

Normally, the lines which describe the relationship between ventricular stroke volume and end-diastolic pressure are as shown in Fig. 1, with 'normal values' marked.

However, with severe RV damage, the RV function curve is shifted downward and to the right. The RV end-diastolic pressure (as assessed by the jugular or CVP) must rise significantly to maintain stroke volume, and may actually exceed LV end-diastolic pressure (or pulmonary capillary wedge pressure) as shown in Fig. 2.

In this case, there is severe RV impairment. The jugular venous pressure has risen hugely, but despite this, RV output is poor. The left ventricle is therefore grossly underfilled despite its normal function. Pre-existing

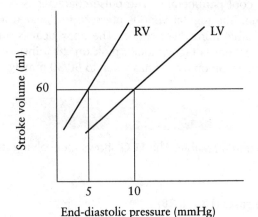

Fig.1 The normal relationship between end-diastolic pressure (EDP) and stroke volume for the left (LV) and right (RV) ventricles. The RVEDP is approximately equivalent to the central venous pressure (CVP), and the LVEDP to the pulmonary artery wedge pressure (PAWP). Note that the LV line is to the right of that for the RV, and slightly downwardly displaced. Thus, at any given stroke volume, the PAWP is normally higher than the CVP.

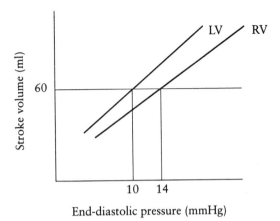

Fig.2 The relationship between end-diastolic pressure (EDP) and stroke volume for the left (LV) and right (RV) ventricles after an RV myocardial infarction. The RV curve is now displaced below and to the right of that for the LV, and CVP is higher than pulmonary artery wedge pressure (PAWP). In other words, the RV now requires a higher filling pressure to maintain the same work (a classic feature of the failing ventricle).

systemic hypertension may have led to LV hypertrophy, and the LV (with diastolic dysfunction) may be more dependent than usual on a high-normal filling pressure.

Cardiogenic shock has ensued, complicated by a metabolic acidosis. Acute renal failure, together with a lactic acidosis from poor tissue perfusion, probably account for both the low arterial pH and the tachypnoea (due to respiratory compensation). There is no evidence of LV failure here, neither clinically, electrocardiographically, nor radiologically.

WHAT TWO DIFFERENTIAL DIAGNOSES SHOULD HAVE RAPIDLY CROSSED YOUR MIND ON FIRST SEEING THE PATIENT?

Hypotension with a raised JVP should immediately trigger thoughts of pulmonary embolus (although massive PE at this stage would be unlikely, as the patient is too well oxygenated), or tamponade (possible after thrombolysis, especially where continuing pain might have suggested myoperi-carditis). The lack of low-voltage ECG trace and pulsus paradoxus, and the readily palpable apex beat are all against this diagnosis, but nonetheless, this diagnosis should be actively excluded as a local posterior collection may yet cause significant dysfunction.

WHAT SHOULD HAVE BEEN SOUGHT ON THE ECG?

The standard 12-lead ECG gives little information about the right ventricle. RV myocardial infarction is best diagnosed using leads $V_1R–V_6R$, which are the mirror (on the right chest) of leads $V_1–V_6$.

ST elevation in lead V_4R alone is more than 80% sensitive and specific for RV myocardial infarction. If ongoing cardiac ischaemia is suspected, always perform right-sided lead recording, and also consider using posterior leads to exclude ongoing posterior ischaemia.

WHAT WOULD THE CORRECT MANAGEMENT HAVE BEEN AT THE REFERRING HOSPITAL IN THE 24 HOURS AFTER HIS PRESENTATION?

Ongoing ischaemia should have been identified using the ECG recordings discussed above. Echocardiography might have suggested RV impairment. The patient should have been referred urgently to the regional cardiology service for immediate angiography and possible angioplasty or revascularization.

HOW ARE YOU GOING TO MANAGE HIS CIRCULATORY STATUS NOW?

Management of RV and LV dysfunction differ. LV support alone without RV support may worsen prognosis.

1. Inotropic support using adrenaline and renal dose dopamine is indicated.
2. Echocardiography should be requested at once to exclude pericardial collection, and to assess RV and LV function.
3. LV filling pressures cannot be inferred from the CVP in this man, and so a pulmonary artery thermodilution catheter should be inserted. A peripheral arterial cannula should also be sited.
4. There is likely to be little RV function, and this ventricle is now little more than a passive conduit. Pulmonary arterial pressure will thus be similar to the CVP. What little RV function remains will depend on a very high filling pressure. Switch off the intravenous nitrates, which will be significantly lowering systemic BP and RV filling pressure. Aggressively fill the patient, whilst repeatedly checking wedge pressure, BP, and cardiac output. You may need CVPs of 30–40 mmHg. Aim to pro-

vide a near-normal pulmonary artery wedge pressure The degree of RV filling required will vary with each case. Initially, filling will raise CVP and cardiac output, and inotropic requirements may fall slightly. However, later on, poor RV compliance will mean that a great rise in CVP increases RV output very little whilst reducing the pressure gradient across the systemic circulation (mean BP–CVP). There is often little further gain in output or perfusion, whilst RV overdistension is detrimental to RV myocardial oxygen supply.

5. Once adequately filled, cardiac output may yet be limited by a high pulmonary vascular resistance. This is not uncommon under such circumstances, and may be due to poor regional lung perfusion and subsequent areas of hypoxic vasoconstriction. A pulmonary vasodilator may be tried, and inhaled nitric oxide (in the ventilated patient) may be highly effective without the dangers of a fall in peripheral vascular resistance. This agent may, in theory, have some beneficial effects on RV function. Prostaglandin infusion into the right atrium may cause vasodilatation in the pulmonary bed more than in the systemic bed. Systemic vasodilators or venodilators should be used with caution. Sudden falls in RV filling pressure or in BP may be catastrophic. Nonetheless, nitrates reintroduced cautiously (with filling to maintain CVP) may increase peripheral perfusion. Phosphodiesterase inhibitors (such as enoximone) may not only act as dilators and inotropes, but also improve RV compliance. Responses to this drug vary wildly in such situations. Start at a low dose, and beware.

6. Call your regional heart transplant unit urgently, and discuss the need for mechanical RV assist device (RVAD). LV support (LV assist device or LVAD) alone worsens prognosis. These supports can be used for many months as a bridge to transplant.

The RV has good collateral support, and it is not unusual to find that myocardial stunning recovers over a fortnight, and RV assistance can be withdrawn. NB. This patient will require haemofiltration to treat his renal failure and to correct his acidosis.

FURTHER READING

Cohn, J. N., Guiha, N. H., Broder, M. I., and Limas, C. J. (1974) Right ventricular infarction. Clinical and haemodynamic features. *Am. J. Cardiol.*, 33, 209–14.

Oldershaw, P. (1992) Assessment of right ventricular function and its role in clinical practice. *Br. Heart J.*, 68, 12–15.

Zehender, M., Kasper, W., Kauder, E., Schonthaler, M., Geibel, A., Olschewski, M., *et al.* (1993) Right ventricular infarction as an independent predictor of prognosis after acute inferior myocardial infarction. *N. Engl. J. Med.*, 328 (14), 981–8.

NOTES

3.5 ENDOCARDITIS

J. B. SALMON MRCP
Consultant Physician
Intensive Care Unit
The Royal Hospital Haslar
Gosport
Hampshire

CASE HISTORY

A 25-year-old man was admitted with a pyrexial illness and confusion. Temperature was 39.5°C; GCS 13; he had a severe digital vasculitis and evidence of mild aortic regurgitation. There were no focal neurological abnormalities and no meningism. Heart rate was 105/min with a normal pulse character and BP was 135/80 mmHg. He had a soft ejection systolic murmur and a short early diastolic murmur of grade 2/4 intensity. A CT brain scan was normal and an echocardiogram showed mild aortic regurgitation with no evidence of vegetations. Blood, urine, and cerebrospinal fluid cultures all yielded a heavy, pure growth of a penicillin-sensitive *Staphylococcus aureus*. A search for obvious sources of infection was negative and there was no history of drug abuse. He was treated with benzylpenicillin, flucloxacillin, and gentamicin but deteriorated acutely 48 hours later. He became hypotensive, breathless, and hypoxaemic such that he required intubation and ventilation.

Initial assessment on the ITU showed a BP of 80/40 mmHg and a 'bounding' pulse at a rate of 125/min. The systolic murmur was unchanged but the diastolic murmur could not be heard. He had crackles throughout both lung fields and a chest X-ray showed a normal cardiac contour with extensive pulmonary oedema.

INVESTIGATIONS

Arterial blood gases (FiO$_2$ 0.7)
PaO_2 8.4 kPa
SBE   −6.5 mmols/l

Pulmonary artery catheterization showed pressures of 45/16 mmHg with a pulmonary artery occlusion pressure of 25 mmHg. Cardiac output by thermodilution was 5 l/min and was not improved by inotropes or cautious colloid challenges.

WHAT HAS CAUSED HIS DETERIORATION?

The original diagnosis includes *S. aureus* aortic endocarditis. This should be considered in all cases of *S. aureus* bacteraemia, especially if there is no obvious primary source, as endocarditis is present in over 40% of such patients. The presence of heart murmurs and digital vasculitis are strong points to the diagnosis. The absence of vegetations on the echocardiogram does not exclude endocarditis. It is difficult to detect vegetations < 3mm in diameter using transthoracic echocardiography. The abrupt deterioration was the result of aortic valve rupture and the key clinical finding was the loss of the aortic diastolic murmur in the context of cardiovascular collapse. This implies that valvar incompetence has become so severe that the pressure gradient across the aortic valve in diastole is negligible. Characteristically, aortic regurgitation leads to a wide pulse pressure with a low diastolic pressure, however both systolic and diastolic pressures may be low when left ventricular failure supervenes. Reviewing this man's observation charts obtained from the ward, showed that there had been a short period during which the BP was 130/50 mmHg in the few hours before he became overtly shocked.

The differential diagnosis includes ARDS. Against this is the high PAOP and the relatively low cardiac output in a patient with hypotension and an apparently hyperdynamic circulation. The patient in fact had a collapsing pulse but this can be difficult to appreciate when the systolic pressure is low.

WHAT IS THE MOST APPROPRIATE INITIAL INVESTIGATION?

He needs an urgent echocardiogram looking not only for evidence of aortic regurgitation but also for evidence of aortic root and septal abscess formation. Transoesophageal echocardiography gives better definition.

WHAT IS THE APPROPRIATE TREATMENT?

He needs urgent aortic valve replacement. Attempts to improve his haemodynamic status by medical management will almost certainly fail and there is no advantage in attempting to control the infection before valve replacement. The mortality of medically-managed endocarditis (all causes) with severe heart failure is approximately 90%, whilst if managed surgically it is 20%. Subsequent prosthetic valve endocarditis occurs in about 10%. Endocarditis is an underdiagnosed condition, a large percentage of cases not being found until post-mortem. The mitral valve is involved most commonly and endocarditis may develop on previously normal valves.

Right-sided endocarditis characteristically occurs in intravenous drug abusers. Increasingly, it is also being recognized as a complication of long-term central venous catheterization. In addition to the characteristic signs of fever, digital vasculitis, and Osler's nodes, other features include a persistently elevated C-reactive protein level and microscopic haematuria. Indications for operation in native valve endocarditis include increasing valvar regurgitation, valve obstruction, left or right ventricular failure, ineffective antimicrobial therapy, myocardial or perivalvar abscess formation, haemodynamically significant septal defects, or fistulae and recurrent emboli. Monitoring of patients who are being managed conservatively should include regular echocardiography to assess valve function and abscess formation. In *S. aureus* endocarditis this should initially be performed daily. Echocardiography in our patient showed severe aortic regurgitation with a dilated left ventricle and a flail aortic right coronary cusp. In theatre, he was found to have extensive abscess formation in the interventricular septum and despite a technically successful operation, died shortly after.

KEY POINTS

1. *S. aureus* bacteraemia shoulde always raise the possibility of endocarditis.
2. In the presence of valvar regurgitation, patients need regular assessment by echocardiography, with early surgical referral if the situation deteriorates.
3. The loss of a documented aortic regurgitant murmur implies worsening of valvar regurgitation, not an improvement.
4. It is difficult to discriminate clinically between a collapsing pulse and a hyperdynamic circulation if the systolic pressure is low.

FURTHER READING

Croft, C. H., Woodward, W., Elliott, A., Commerford, P. J., Barnard, C. N., and Beck, W. (1983) Analysis of surgical versus medical therapy in active complicated native valve endocarditis. *Am. J. Cardiol.* 51, 1650–5.

Griffin, F. M., Jones, G., Cobbs, G. (1972) Aortic insufficiency in bacterial endocarditis. *Ann. Intern. Med.*, 76, 23–8.

Kereiakes, D. J. and Porto, T. A. (1987) Emergencies in vascular heart disease. In (ed. B. H. Greenberg and G. Murphy) Valvular heart disease, pp. 215–33 PSG Publishing, Littleton, MA.

Mugge, A., Daniel, W. G., Frank, G., and Lichten, P. R. (1989) Echocardiography in infective endocarditis: reassessment of prognostic implications of vegetation size determined by the transthoracic and the transoesophageal approach. *J. Am. Coll. Cardiol.*, 14, 631–8.

NOTES

3.6 HEART BLOCK

D. Rosser MRCP FRCA
Consultant Physician, Intensive Care Unit
University Hospital
Birmingham

CASE HISTORY

You are asked to see a 58-year-old lady on the cardiac surgical ICU who has recurrent ventricular fibrillation. You are told that she has had an aortic valve replacement that day which was uneventful, although she has marked left ventricular hypertrophy. She was otherwise well preoperatively except for controlled hypertension. Postoperatively she was noted to have become bradycardic, rate 40/min, shortly before going into ventricular tachycardia which rapidly regenerated to ventricular fibrillation. She responded to a 220 J DC shock, emerging into a broad complex bradycardia of 40/min with a BP of 95/40 mmHg (MAP 55 mmHg) for some minutes before again degenerating to ventricular tachycardia/fibrillation (VT/VF). This sequence of events was repeated twice more despite the administration of 100 mg of lignocaine intravenously. Prior to her first arrest she was ventilated with good blood gases, normal acid-base status, and blood biochemistry.

The attending doctor felt that the recurrent VT/VF was due to the slow underlying heart rate and administered atropine and then isoprenaline. The patient then went into VF for a fourth time, from which, despite a further 75 mg of lignocaine, she was only resuscitated after a number of DC shocks over a period of 15 minutes.

On arrival you find the patient with a BP of 84/36 mmHg and a heart rate of 54/min on an isoprenaline infusion. She has a broad complex irregular rhythm with at least three different QRS complex morphologies seen.

WHAT IS THE LIKELY UNDERLYING PROBLEM AND PATHOPHYSIOLOGICAL EXPLANATION FOR THIS PREDISPOSITION TO RECURRENT TACHYDYSRHYTHMIAS?

Complete heart block is the likely underlying rhythm, being common after aortic surgery. A patient with significant left ventricular hypertrophy will be unable to compensate for the decrease in heart rate by increasing stroke volume (cardiac output = heart rate × stroke volume) because of the decreased compliance of the ventricle. This leads to a decrease in cardiac output and thus to hypotension. Furthermore, a hypertrophied ventricle requires a higher than normal perfusion pressure to achieve adequate coronary perfusion, especially in the presence of pre-existing hypertension. Thus the hypotension associated with bradycardias in these patients induces a vicious spiral with decreasing myocardial perfusion, impairing left ventricular function and predisposing to arrhythmias which in turn exacerbate the hypotension.

WHICH PART OF THE TREATMENT HAS EXACERBATED THE PROBLEM AND HOW HAS IT DONE SO?

The administration of atropine and isoprenaline has exacerbated the problem. These agents are given in order to increase heart rate. However, the potential increase in the intrinsic rate of the ventricle (the pacemaker in complete heart block) is modest. The positive effect on BP brought about by the increase in heart rate-induced improvement in cardiac output is more than offset by the vasodilatation induced by both atropine and particularly, isoprenaline. Thus despite improving heart rate these agents often further lower the BP, exacerbating the myocardial hypoperfusion and irritability. In addition, both drugs pre-dispose to ventricular tachy-dysrhthmias by their mode of action.

WHAT SHOULD HAVE BEEN DONE AND HOW MAY IT BE ACHIEVED?

The treatment of complete heart block is by temporary pacing, not by pharmacological methods. Patients recovering from cardiac surgery often have ventricular pacing wires placed during the operation. Other techniques include transcutaneous pacing devices which can be operated quickly and simply through pads placed on the front and back of the chest, or transvenous pacing which can be established using either a traditional X-ray screened wire or a balloon flotation wire.

IF THE TREATMENT OF CHOICE IS NOT IMMEDIATELY POSSIBLE, WHAT PHARMACOLOGICAL TREATMENT WOULD HAVE BEEN MORE APPROPRIATE THAN THAT WHICH SHE RECEIVED?

If necessary, an agent such as adrenaline with chronotropic and vasopressor effects is more appropriate in the short term while pacing is established as this will maintain BP and thus myocardial perfusion. The increase in myocardial perfusion will more than offset the intrinsic arrhythmogenic tendencies of adrenaline.

FURTHER READING

Eckstein, J. W. and Abboud, F. M. (1962) Circulatory effects of sympathomimetic amines. *Am. Heart J.*, **63**, 119–35.

Edhag, O. and Swahn, A. (1976) Prognosis of patients with complete heart block or arrhythmic syncope who were not treated with artificial pacemakers. *Acta. Med. Scand.*, **200**, 457–63.

Sainsbury, E. J., Fitzpatrick, D., Ikram, H., Nicholls, M. G., Espiner, E. A., and Ashley, J. J. (1985) Pharmacokinetics and plasma-concentration-effect relationships of prenalterol in cardiac failure. *Eur. J. Clin. Pharmacol.*, **28**, 397–403.

NOTES

Part 4 Infection

4.1 TUBERCULOSIS

S. G. Spiro MD FRCP
Consultant Physician
Middlesex Hospital
UCL
London

CASE HISTORY

A 24-year-old Sierra Leonese lady was admitted to hospital with a 1-week history of increasing dyspnoea, fever, cough, and no sputum. Her last menstrual period was 3 months ago as she had had a Caesarian section and was breast-feeding her baby. She entered the United Kingdom to live with her cousin also 3 months ago. She was single and was previously healthy. She was on no medication and did not appear to be on any drugs of addiction.

EXAMINATION FINDINGS

On admission she was ill, breathless, confused, and uncooperative (for 2 days). Core temperature 38°C; BP 100/70 mmHg; pulse 100/min.

INVESTIGATIONS

Urea and electrolytes:	normal
Alk. phosphatase	460 iu/l
Bilirubin	30 μmol/l
Gamma GT	36 iu/l
AST	122 iu/l
Hb	11.2 g/dl
WCC	12.1×10^9/l (68% neutrophils)
Platelets	125×10^9/l

Arterial blood gases

PaO_2	8 kPa
$PaCO_2$	3.6 kPa
pH	7.35

Chest X-ray: extensive bilateral basal and midzone confluent shadowing, typical of ARDS

WHAT IS THE LIKELY DIAGNOSIS? DISCUSS MANAGEMENT AND TREATMENT

The patient has presented with a clinical syndrome of ARDS. The likely causes considered initially were:

1 Drug abuse – no evidence of this from relatives;
2 Bacterial sepsis secondary to pneumonia – the lack of a high WCC and normal blood cultures in a patient not taking antibiotics made this less likely, although broad spectrum intravenous antibiotics were commenced;
3 Pelvic sepsis – a pregnancy test was negative and there was no evidence of retained products. Her operation scar was well-healed.

The history of malaise along with entry from a country with a moderate incidence of tuberculosis (TB) made this a possible cause of the lung disorder. There were HIV risk factors (possible TB and sub-Saharan African origin) but HIV I and II antibodies were negative.

The patient's condition deteriorated despite intravenous antibiotics and, on day two, she required intubation and mechanical ventilation. Fibre-optic bronchoscopy and lavage of the right middle lobe found no pathogens and was negative for acid fast bacteria (AFB) on direct smear. A liver biopsy and bone marrow culture/trephine biopsy were taken. The liver biopsy showed multiple non-caseating granulomata and AFB was seen on ZN staining of the bone marrow.

Disseminated TB (acute miliary TB) is rare, but has a very serious prognosis with an up to 88% mortality. Rarely, as in this patient, TB may present as acute respiratory failure and can cause a clinical and radiological picture of ARDS with a very rapid onset from a previously normal chest X-ray in days. Occasionally the diagnosis is hampered by co-existing bacterial super-infection. In some cases of this type of presentation, sputum is smear positive for AFB. If negative, broncho-alveolar lavage at fibre-optic bronchoscopy is potentially useful although the incidence of a positive direct smear in miliary TB is low.

A trans-bronchial lung biopsy in a patient already mechanically ventilated, or hypoxic and likely to require mechanical ventilation, is dangerous because of the possibility of a pneumothorax. However, even though it is likely to produce a diagnosis and is probably the procedure of choice, it was not attempted in this case. Liver biopsy and bone marrow aspirate and trephine were preferred, and in fact provided the prognosis.

It is important to emphasize that the diagnosis of TB can be difficult and should be intensively looked for if it is considered a possibility. The diagnostic role of the polymerase chain reaction (PCR) in the evaluation of active TB is still uncertain, i.e. a positive reaction may not necessarily mean current active disease. The prognosis worsens the longer the delay before treatment is commenced. Nevertheless, in up to 80% of cases, the diagnosis is only established at autopsy. The disadvantage of liver and marrow biopsy is that the diagnosis is rarely made on direct smear examination, but on cultures which take 4–8 weeks. The incidence of granulomata in the liver, is up to 80% in advanced TB and can be considered diagnostic in the appropriate clinical setting. Sarcoidosis and other causes of granulomata would not present in this manner.

Conventional anti-tuberculous therapy is given for miliary TB, i.e. rifampicin, isoniazid, and pyrazinamide. Despite no clear data conferring an advantage for the addition of cortico-steroids, they were given to this patient – in a high dose of 400 mg hydrocortisone, intravenously, 6-hourly – because of the enzyme-inducing effects of rifampicin. Although the addition of isoniazid and pyrazinamide to rifampicin does not increase the risk of hepatitis as an important side-effect to this therapy, hepatitis occurs more frequently if the liver function is abnormal when treatment is initiated. A transient rise of liver enzymes is expected during the early weeks of therapy, but the serum values rarely more than double. In our patient, the enzymes rose progressively, the alkaline phosphatase exceeded 1000 iu/l after two weeks of therapy and the bilirubin rose to 90 μmol/l, causing therapy to be withdrawn. The management of this complication involves cessation of all three of these potentially hepato-toxic drugs until the bilirubin and liver enzymes return to normal. It is then safe to resume all three drugs in normal doses as the hepatic damage does not recur. It is probably safe to stop anti-tuberculous therapy for the month or so that the liver requires to recover, provided 2 weeks of triple therapy has been given, i.e. sufficient to kill a high percentage of the tubercle bacilli. However, data on the safety of a significant gap in therapy in a seriously-ill patient is lacking and, in our patient, intramuscular streptomycin and oral ethambutol per nasogastric tube were substituted.

KEY POINTS

Tuberculosis is a rare, but important, cause of ARDS and should be considered in any patient who has lived in a country with a high prevalence of the disease. It is commoner in patients on immuno-suppressive treatment, especially if the chest X-ray shows evidence of old (untreated) TB, or if the patient has a chronic immuno-suppressive disease or malignancy.

FURTHER READING

Piqueras, A. R., Marruecos, L., Artigas, A., and Rodriguez, C. (1987) Miliary tuberculosis and the adult respiratory distress syndrome. *Intensive Care Med.*, 13, 175–82.

Sydow, M., Schauer, A., Crozier, T. A., and Bucchard, I. H. (1992) Multiple organ failure in generalized disseminated tuberculosis. *Resp. Med.*, 86, 517–19.

NOTES

4.2 HUMAN IMMUNODEFICIENCY VIRUS (HIV)

A. Severn PhD MRCP
Staff Grade Physician, In-Patient HIV/AIDS Unit
and
R. F. Miller FRCP
Senior Lecturer, Division of Pathology and Infectious Diseases,
UCL Medical School; Consultant Physician, Camden and Islington
Community Health Services (NHS) Trust
Middlesex Hospital
London

CASE HISTORY

A 32-year-old caucasian, homosexual, male teacher was admitted to a general medical ward with a 4-week history of increasing exertional dyspnoea and unproductive cough. He had been HIV-I antibody positive for 6 years and his most recent CD4 lymphocyte count was $0.22 \times 10^9/1$ (normal range $= 0.35 -2.2 \times 10^9/l$). He had no previous AIDS defining diagnoses and was taking no prophylaxis against *Pneumocystis carinii* pneumonia (PCP).

EXAMINATION FINDINGS

On examination he was centrally cyanosed, tachypnoeic (36 breaths per minute), and pyrexial. Temperature 37.8°C. There were no abnormalities in the mouth or on the skin.

INVESTIGATIONS

A chest radiograph showed diffuse bilateral interstitial shadowing.

Arterial blood gases (FiO$_2$ 0.6)

PaO$_2$	7.2 kPa
PaCO$_2$	4.6 kPa
pH	7.31
HCO$_3$	19 mmol/l
Saturation	86%

DISCUSS MANAGEMENT AND TREATMENT

The history is strongly suggestive of PCP and specific treatment for this condition should be started empirically. Fibreoptic bronchoscopy would be hazardous in this situation. The patient has severe disease (prolonged respiratory symptoms greater than 3 weeks duration, tachypnoea, a severely abnormal chest radiograph, and marked arterial hypoxaemia) and so should be given high-dose intravenous co-trimoxazole (20 mg/kg per day of trimethoprim component in divided doses) and steroids (methyl-prednisolone 1 g intravenously once-daily for 3 days, then 0.5 g once-daily for 2 days, followed by a tapering course of oral prednisolone 60 mg→nil. over 10 days). If the patient is allergic to co-trimoxazole then intravenous pentamidine (4 mg/kg once daily) may be given with methyl-prednisolone. Response to pentamidine (4–7 days) is slower than to co-trimoxazole (3–5 days). Nebulized pentamidine, or oral atovoquone, dapsone/trimethoprim, or clindamyacin/primaquine should not be used as these regimens are of no proven benefit in PCP of this severity.

As oxygenation is poor, despite a high FiO_2, a trial of mask (or nasal) CPAP is indicated. There is a significant risk of pneumothorax if > 7.5 cmH_2O of PEEP is used. It may be necessary to use an FiO_2 of 1.0 in order to maintain oxygenation. A failed trial of CPAP is an indication for intubation and mechanical ventilation. Mechanical ventilation should always be considered in first episode PCP. It is important to take into account the wishes of the patient and his partner/next of kin.

Mask CPAP (FiO_2 0.85, PEEP 5 cmH_2O) was commenced on admission to ICU, together with intravenous co-trimoxazole and methylprednisolone. Hypoxaemia persisted, PaO_2 8.1 kPa and tachypnoea increased with a respiratory rate of 30/min. The patient was intubated 4 hours after admission to ICU, but died 36 hours later from a cardiac arrest secondary to refractory hypoxaemia.

KEY POINTS

1. PCP remains a common cause of severe pneumonia in HIV-positive patients.
2. Adjunctive glucocorticoids given to patients with moderate or severe PCP significantly reduce the need for mechanical ventilation and mortality. The most benefit is seen if steroids are begun with specific antimicrobial therapy. Thus, in some patients it may be necessary to begin steroid and empirical antimicrobial therapy without a firm diagnosis.
3. In those failing a trial of CPAP who are mechanically ventilated, mortality is high (> 50% if deterioration occurs within a few days of treatment, and almost 100% if deterioration occurs after a week or more of antimicrobial therapy).
4. It is important to note that PCP *per se* may produce a clinical syndrome which is indistinguishable from Gram-negative sepsis with high cardiac output, low systemic vascular resistance, and low BP.

FURTHER READING

Jeffrey, A. A., Bullen, C., and Miller, R. F. (1993) Intensive care management of severe *Pneumocystis carinii* pneumonia. *Care Crit. Ill*, 9, 258–60.

Miller, R. F. (1994) Prophylaxis and treatment of *Pneumocystis carinii* pneumonia. *Drug and Thera. Bull.*, 32, 12–15.

Miller, R. F. and Mitchell, D. (1995) *Pneumocystis carinii* pneumonia. *Thorax*, 50, 191–200.

Miller, R. F. and Semple, S. J. G. (1991) Continuous positive airway pressure ventilation for respiratory failure associated with *Pneumocystis carinii* pneumonia. *Respiratory Med.*, 85, 133–8.

NOTES

4.3 LEPTOSPIROSIS

D. G. SINCLAIR MD MRCP
Consultant Physician
Torbay General Hospital
Devon

CASE HISTORY

A previously-well, 22-year-old male was brought to casualty as an emergency. On admission he gave a history of a pyrexial illness of 3 days duration. There was no history of foreign travel or drug ingestion.

EXAMINATION FINDINGS

Positive findings on examination were marked jaundice; temperature 38°C; a small right-sided inferior subconjunctival haemorrhage; the liver was just palpable; the musculature of both legs was swollen and exquisitely tender; cerebration was sluggish; and he was mildly confused. BP was 120/60 mmHg; pulse 110/min; respiratory rate 20/min. Catheterization of the bladder revealed a small quantity of urine.

INVESTIGATIONS

Biochemistry

Sodium	130 mmol/l
Potassium	6.3 mmol/l
Urea	40 mmol/l
Creatinine	626 μmol/l
Bilirubin	230 μmol/l
ALT	303 iu/l
Creatine kinase	11 141 iu/l
Prothrombin time	20 secs

Arterial blood gases

PaO_2	8.2 kPa
$PaCO_2$	2.9 kPa
pH	7.53

Urine

SG	1010
Blood	++++
Protein	++++

DISCUSS DIFFERENTIAL DIAGNOSIS AND MANAGEMENT

This young man is suffering from respiratory and hepatorenal failure. The history of a pyrexial illness with myalgia, rhabdomyolysis, subconjunctival haemorrhage, and hepatorenal failure are strong pointers towards a diagnosis of leptospirosis. This infectious disease is caused by one of the serotypes of the spirochaete Leptospira. In mild cases the disease may be subclinical. Severe infections such as this, with jaundice and renal failure, are known as Weil's disease.

Immediate management should address the patient's hypoxia, fluid status and exclude an obstructive cause for the renal failure. Arterial and CVP monitoring should be performed following placement of appropriate cannulae. A chest X-ray should be carried out in an attempt to establish the cause of the respiratory failure and exclude pulmonary oedema. An abdominal ultrasound scan should be undertaken to examine the hepatic parenchyma, biliary and renal tracts, and in the absence of urinary tract obstruction the CVP should cautiously be challenged, using small aliquots of colloid fluid until a sustained rise of 3 cmH$_2$O is achieved. If normalization of CVP has no effect on urine output, intravenous frusemide in a dose of up to 250 mg given over 15 minutes may be tried. If there is no response to these measures, in the presence of hyperkalaemia and a rising urea, renal replacement therapy should be commenced early. Ideally this should be undertaken using haemofiltration or dialysis. Peritoneal dialysis may also be employed, although clearly this is not ideal for a patient with respiratory failure.

Leptospirosis remains uncommon in the UK. The disease is transmitted from animals to humans via contamination of soil and water by infected animal urine. The usual portal of entry are abrasions on the skin and exposed conjunctival, nasal, and oral mucus membranes, the normal incubation period being 7–13 days. The main occupations at risk are farm-workers and those undertaking fresh-water activities, e.g. windsurfing and river-rafting.

Leptospirosis causes a widespread vasculitis with the subsequent development of myositis, pneumonitis, peritonitis, nephritis, meningitis, carditis, gastritis, and conjunctivitis. The diagnosis can be rapidly confirmed by the Public Health Laboratory using an immunoglobulin M-specific enzyme-linked immunosorbent assay and a genus specific microscopic agglutination test. Treatment of affected organ systems is supportive. Although the beneficial role of antimicrobial agents in human leptospirosis is controversial, most investigators agree that penicillin or tetracycline should be given as early in the course of the disease as possible to maximize any potential benefit. Most patients survive with good recovery of renal function.

KEY POINTS

1. Consider the diagnosis of leptospirosis in cases of acute renal and hepatorenal failure, particularly in patients who indulge in water sports.
2. In cases of acute renal failure consider early institution of renal replacement therapy.

FURTHER READING

Watkins, S. A. (1985). Update on leptospirosis. *Br. Med. J.* **290**, 1502–3.

Watt, G., Tuazon, M. L., Santiago, E., *et al.* (1988). Placebo-controlled trial of intravenous penicillin for severe and late leptospirosis. *Lancet*, i, 433–5.

NOTES

4.4 LEGIONNAIRES' DISEASE

G. L. RIDGWAY MD MRCP FRCPATH.

Consultant Microbiologist
UCL Hospitals
London

CASE HISTORY

A 64-year-old chronic bronchitic consulted his GP complaining of increasing dyspnoea, and a cough producing yellow sputum. He smoked 15–20 cigarettes daily, and drank 20 units of alcohol per week. It was noted that he kept a budgerigar. The GP prescribed oral amoxycillin. 36 hours later he was referred to hospital as he had become peripherally cyanotic, severely dyspnoeic at rest, and mentally confused.

EXAMINATION FINDINGS

Oral temperature 38.5°C; tachypnoea (30/min). Percussive dullness both lung fields, widespread crackles, and patchy bronchial breathing. Pulse 110/min., irregularly irregular. Palpable liver edge.

INVESTIGATIONS

Biochemistry

Hb	15.2 g/dl
WCC	13.9×10^9/l
Sodium	129 mmol/l
Potassium	3.1 mmol/l
Urea	24.3 mmol/l
Creatinine	561 μmols/l
Protein	56 g/l
Albumin	27 g/l
Bilirubin	73 μmols/l
AST	67 iu/l
Alkaline phosphatase	57 iu/l
Glucose	6.3 mmol/l

Arterial blood gases (FiO$_2$ 0.6)

PaO$_2$	8 kPa
PaCO$_2$	6.6 kPa
Urine:	protein and bilirubin present

Chest X-ray: Left lower lobe pneumonia with patchy consolidation of right, mid, and lower zones

DISCUSS MANAGEMENT AND TREATMENT. WHAT MICROBIOLOGICAL INVESTIGATIONS WILL YOU INSTIGATE?

The patient falls into the high mortality group as identified in the British Thoracic Society Guidelines (Age > 60 years; diastolic blood pressure < 60 mmHg; respiratory rate > 30/min; atrial fibrillation; confused; urea > 7 mmol/l; arterial oxygen tension < 8 kPa; WCC > 20 or < 4 × 10^9/l; albumin < 53 g/l; multiple lobes affected on CXR). He therefore requires admission to the ICU. In addition to the obvious severe pneumonia, the patient has renal failure, evidence of hepatic dysfunction, and clouding of consciousness. There is mild hyponatraemia. This involvement of several organ systems is suggestive of an atypical pneumonia but similar findings can accompany severe pneumococcal infection and differentiation on clinical grounds can be very difficult. The history of keeping a budgerigar raises the possibility of psittacosis. However, this is rare in the UK and having established that the bird is not recently purchased and is fit, this diagnosis is unlikely.

Initial management is standard for any patient with severe pneumonia: high concentration oxygen therapy with intubation and ventilation (if required), attention to the circulation, and consideration of renal support. The antibiotic depends on the setting in which the pneumonia was acquired. This pneumonia is, by definition, community-acquired, and, therefore, irrespective of the likely aetiology, the initial chemotherapy should be empirical. The current recommendation is for a parenteral 2nd generation cephalosporin, or a non-anti pseudomonal 3rd generation cephalosporin (e.g. cefuroxime, cefotaxime, ceftriaxone), plus a macrolide (e.g. erythromycin). It should be noted that failure to respond to a β lactam antibiotic (in this case, amoxycillin), coupled with the non-specific involvement of the other systems, is suggestive of an 'atypical' pneumonia (i.e. one that does not respond to standard β lactam therapy). Initially, it is prudent to continue the combination therapy. Quinolones (e.g. ciprofloxacin) should not be used as first-line therapy because of uncertainty concerning their activity against pneumococci.

Failure of the patient to respond to the antibiotics, particularly if multisystem disorders increase, or positive evidence of *Legionella* spp. infection is available, should lead to the substitution of the cephalosporin by rifampicin, the macrolide being continued in addition. The resolution of all atypical pneumonias is often prolonged.

AETIOLOGY OF COMMUNITY ACQUIRED PNEUMONIA

Common – *Streptococcus pneumoniae, Mycoplasma pneumoniae.*
Less common – Respiratory viruses, *Haemophilus influenzae, Chlamydia pneumoniae, Legionella* spp.
Rare – *Staphylococcus aureus*, Gram-negative aerobic rods, Anaerobes, *Chlamydia psittaci, Coxiella burnetti.*

Up to 30% of patients with pneumococcal disease will be bacteraemic, hence the importance of the blood culture. In this case, prior chemotherapy, particularly with a β lactam, reduces the chances of isolating the organism. Sputum examination is frequently unhelpful. An urgent microscopy may assist if the specimen is frankly purulent, particularly if the aetiology is pneumococcal, the much rarer staphylococcal or klebsiella pneumonias. Sputum microscopy will only rarely result in a change of therapy. Sputum culture is also often unhelpful, even when a potential pathogen is isolated, owing to the possibility of upper respiratory tract colonization. The laboratory attempts to circumvent this problem by digesting and diluting the sputum before culture. The results are not entirely satisfactory. Routine sputum culture does not usually include cultures for *Legionella* spp. If the suspicion is strong, the laboratory must be contacted, and charcoal yeast-extract agar cultures set up. Direct immunofluorescent antigen tests for *Legionella* spp. and *Chlamydia pneumoniae* are generally unreliable, and not widely available. A clotted blood sample should be screened for IgM antibody against *Mycoplasma pneumoniae*, using gelatin particle agglutination, as this test is positive early in the disease (the presence of cold agglutinins is a useful but non-specific test for mycoplasma infection). The residual serum should be saved.

Other serological tests should not be requested at this time, as they are unlikely to be of help, and may mislead. A second sample of serum will be required at least 14 days later, and tested for antibody to *Legionella* spp. (rapid micro agglutination test (RMAT), immunofluorescent antibody test (IFAT), *Chlamydia pneumoniae, C. psittaci*, whole inclusion immuno-fluorescence test (WIF), and complement fixation test (CFT). Antibodies to *Legionella* spp., and *Chlamydia pneumoniae* may not appear for several weeks, often requiring examination of a third serum sample to exclude the diagnosis. Urine enzyme-linked immunosorbent assay (ELISA) for *Legionella* spp. antigen may be available via a reference laboratory, and is positive early in the disease. Negative findings do not exclude the disease.

This patient had acute pneumonia caused by *Legionella pneumophilia* serogroup 1. The source of the infection was a building with a contaminated cooling tower. There were several other associated cases.

FURTHER READING

British Thoracic Society. (1991) Guidelines for the management of community-acquired pneumonia in adults admitted to hospital. *Br. J. Hosp. Med.*, **49**, 346–50.

Hosker, H. S. R., Jones, G. M., and Hawkey, P. (1994) Management of community-acquired lower respiratory tract infection. *Br. Med. J.*, **308**, 701–5.

Winn, W. C. (1988) Legionnaire's disease: historical perspective. *Clin. Microbiol. Rev.*, **1**, 60–81.

4.5 MALARIA

J. F. DOHERTY MD MRCP DTM&H
and
P. L. CHIODINI PhD FRCP
The Hospital for Tropical Diseases
London

CASE HISTORY

A 31-year-old woman was found unconscious at home 13 days after returning from a holiday in Zambia. At presentation, she was febrile 39°C, jaundiced, and dehydrated with a disconjugate gaze. She was flexing in response to painful stimuli and had generalized muscle twitching. She had generalized hypertonia without localizing signs. There was no hepatosplenomegaly. She weighed 70 kg.

INVESTIGATIONS

Biochemistry

Hb	12.6 gm/dl
WCC	11.8×10^9/l
Platelets	14×10^9/l
Sodium	137 mmols/l
Potassium	5.8 mmols/l
Urea	27.0 mmols/l
Creatinine	370 μmols/l

Arterial blood gases

PaO_2	14.8 kPa
$PaCO_2$	2.3 kPa
pH	7.29

Malaria parasite screen revealed trophozoites and schizonts of *Plasmodium falciparum* with a parasitaemia of 21% in the peripheral blood

DISCUSS MANAGEMENT AND TREATMENT

Drug treatment

Quinine remains the drug of choice for *Plasmodium falciparum* malaria. The dosage is 10 mg/kg body weight (to a maximum of 600 mg) of quinine dihydrochloride (for parenteral therapy) or quinine sulphate (for oral therapy). The chosen route depends on the clinical condition of the patient. In this case, the patient had pyrexia of 39°C, evidence of cerebral and renal involvement, thrombocytopenia, and a very high parasitaemia in the peripheral blood. In addition, the presence of schizonts (the last stage of the erythrocytic cycle) In the peripheral blood implies a heavy infection and the possibility of a rapid increase in the parasitaemia. She was therefore given intravenous quinine dihydrochloride 600 mg in 250 ml of normal saline over 4 hours. The timing of further dosages in such severely-ill patients are best managed by regular measurement of plasma quinine concentration.

A loading dose infusion of 20 mg/kg body weight should be given in cases of severe malaria in children and in adults who acquire severe falciparum malaria in south-east Asia. The necessity for a loading dose in adults with malaria acquired in Africa remains an open question.

Exchange blood transfusion has been advocated in patients with complicated malaria and high peripheral parasitaemia, although no controlled trial has been performed. This patient received a 6 unit exchange through a double-lumen Vascath inserted in the femoral vein.

Once the parasites have cleared from the peripheral blood, a second agent should be given to reduce the risk of recurrence. Options include Fansidar (pyrimethamine/sulphadoxine), mefloquine, or doxycycline, with the choice depending on the geographical history.

Recently, two preliminary studies have reported additional benefit from adjunctive therapy with desferrioxamine (an iron-chelating agent) and pentoxifylline (an inhibitor of tumour necrosis factor).

Adjunctive therapy

Acute tubular necrosis (ATN) is a well-recognized complication of severe malaria. In addition, high output cardiac failure and acute respiratory distress syndrome (ARDS) may develop, particularly in adults. Fluid overload is particularly dangerous in malaria and careful management of fluid balance is therefore essential. If an exchange transfusion is performed, it must be isovolumetric. This patient had a Swan Ganz catheter inserted under platelet cover, received 3.5 l of fluid in the first 24 hours, and was then managed with neutral fluid balance. Rehydration, haemofiltration, and haemodialysis may all be necessary. The role of bicarbonate remains controversial.

Lactic acidosis correlates with prognosis in patients with malaria.

Generalized grand mal convulsions are common among patients with cerebral malaria, particularly children. Diazepam should be used in the first instance, followed by phenytoin or phenobarbitone. Some authors recommend prophylactic anti-convulsants for all patients with cerebral malaria.

Hypoglycaemia may occur in any patient with severe malaria but is particularly likely in patients receiving parenteral quinine. Quinine is thought to stimulate insulin release from the pancreatic beta-cells. Close monitoring of blood sugar is therefore mandatory.

KEY POINTS

1. Quinine is the drug of choice for *P. falciparum* malaria.
2. Renal failure, ARDS, convulsions, and hypoglycaemia are well-recognized complications of malaria.

FURTHER READING

Di Perri, G., *et al.* (1995) Pentoxifylline as a supportive agent in the treatment of cerebral malaria. *J.Infect.Dis.*, **171**, 1317–22.

Gordeuk, V., *et al.* (1992) Effect of iron chelation on recovery from deep coma in children with cerebral malaria. *N.Engl.J.Med.*, **327**:1473–7.

Warrell, D. A., Molyneux, M. E., and Beales, P. F. (1990) Severe and complicated malaria. *Trans.R.Soc. Trop.Med.Hyg.*, **84** (2), 1–65.

NOTES

T. DAVIDSON Ch.M. MRCP FRCS
Department of Surgery
UCL Hospitals
London

CASE HISTORY

A 62-year-old male is admitted via the A&E department with an 8-hour history of severe increasing upper abdominal pain. The pain radiates from the epigastrium through into the back and is associated with nausea and retching. The patient has not had previous similar episodes and there is no history of abdominal surgery or drug ingestion.

EXAMINATION FINDINGS

He is tachycardic; pulse 110/min; respiratory rate 30/min; BP 100/65 mmHg. Clammy peripheries and upper abdominal peritonism. Sweating and distressed, but not jaundiced.

INVESTIGATIONS

Biochemistry		Arterial blood gases (on room air)	
Sodium	132 mmol/l	PaO_2	8.2 kPa
Potassium	4.2 mmol/l	$PaCO_2$	3.4 kPa
Urea	12 mmol/l	pH	7.32
Creatinine	140 μmol/l		
Amylase	1100 iu/l		
Hb	16.2 g/dl		
WCC	$18.7 \times 10^9/l$		
Platelets	$280,000 \times 10^9/l$		

Urine: concentrated appearance, ketones 2+, glucose 1+ Blood: trace.

DISCUSS THESE RESULTS AND OUTLINE THE
MANAGEMENT, WITH PARTICULAR REFERENCE
TO THE INDICATIONS FOR ENDOSCOPIC
RETROGRADE CHOLANGIOPANCREATOGRAPHY
(ERCP) AND FOR SURGERY IN THE FACE OF
CONTINUING CLINICAL DETERIORATION

In this clinical setting the serum amylase of 1100 iu/l is diagnostic of acute pancreatitis. The actual level of amylase bears no relationship to the severity of the pancreatitis which is assessed on clinical and other biochemical criteria. In this patient, tachycardia, tachypnoea, and hypotension are poor prognostic signs. The hypoxaemia on admission likewise indicates severe systemic decompensation and can explain the hypocarbia from hyperventilation. There is also hypovolaemia and a metabolic acidosis with compensatory hyperventilation in this patient. Other Ranson's criteria of severe acute pancreatitis on admission are age > 55, blood glucose > 10 mmol/l, LDH > 300 iu/l, SGOT > 250 iu/l, WCC $> 16 \times 10^9/l$.

Most attacks of acute pancreatitis are self-limiting. Management comprises supportive treatment, requiring ITU admission in severe cases, as well as investigations to establish the cause of the pancreatitis.

Fluid replacement is the most important requirement in the early treatment of pancreatitis. In severe pancreatitis, CVP monitoring and urinary catheterization are mandatory. Where large fluid shifts occur, measurements of cardiac output and pulmonary capillary occlusion pressure may be necessary, especially if cardiac or renal compromise develop. Hypoxaemia is common in acute pancreatitis and in the early stages occurs without chest radiographic abnormality. With disease progression hypoxaemia may accompany atelectasis, pleural effusions, diaphragmatic elevation, pulmonary oedema, and late respiratory failure secondary to systemic sepsis.

Respiratory support with oxygen, humidification of airways, ventilatory exercise, and occasionally mechanical ventilation are required. Minimizing pancreatic secretion is achieved by bowel rest, nasogastric intubation and regular aspiration, and H_2 receptor blockers. Treatment with antiprotease and anticholinergic agents are not of proven benefit. In severe pancreatitis where tissue necrosis is likely, there is a risk of secondary bacterial infection and prophylactic broad spectrum antibiotics are justified.

Intervention in the form of ERCP and sphincterotomy has a role in severe gall stone pancreatitis. Early abdominal ultrasound is indicated to establish the presence of gall stones. There is evidence that early ERCP and endoscopic sphincterotomy is of benefit in this clinical setting. An experienced endoscopist is required to minimize major potential complications from this procedure. There is consensus that ERCP confers no benefit in severe alcoholic pancreatitis nor in mild pancreatitis from any etiology.

Peritoneal lavage remains controversial in the early phase of acute pancreatitis. Some studies have shown benefit when there is early major plasma volume loss, persistent hypotension, or continued clinical deterioration. Lavage is performed via a dialysis catheter and the purpose is to wash out the ascitic fluid and its toxins (kinins and other vasoactive amines such as kallikrein and bradykinin). Continued deterioration after the first 4 or 5 days may be due to pancreatic and peri-pancreatic necrosis with liquefaction and secondary infection in rare cases. Percutaneous drainage may be effective in a single cavity, but surgery is required for debridement of extensive necrotic and septic retroperitoneal tissues.

KEY POINTS

1. Most attacks of pancreatitis are mild, self-limiting and can be managed on the general surgical or medical ward.
2. If an experienced endoscopist is available, early ERCP/sphincterotomy is indicated in severe gallstone pancreatitis.
3. Laparotomy is occasionally required for debridement of necrotic tissue in the desperately-ill patient.

FURTHER READING

Fan, S. T., Lai, E., Mok, F. P. T., Lo, C. M., Zheng, S. S., and Wong, J. (1993) Early treatment of acute biliary pancreatitis by endoscopic papillotomy. *N.Engl.J.Med.*, **328**, 228–32.

Neoptolemos, J. P., Carr-Locke, D. L., London, N. J., Bailey, I. A., James, D., and Fossard, D. P. (1988) Controlled trial of urgent endoscopic retrograde cholangiopancreatography and endoscopic sphincterotomy versus conservative treatment for acute pancreatitis due to gallstones. *Lancet*, **8618**, 980–3.

Ratner, D. W. and Warshaw, A. L. (1991) Acute pancreatitis. In (ed. P. J. Morris and M. Malt) *Oxford textbook of surgery*, pp. 1289–98. Oxford University Press, Oxford.

NOTES

4.7 SEPSIS

C. J. HINDS FRCP FRCA

Senior Lecturer in Intensive Care and Anaesthesia
The Medical College of St Bartholomew's Hospital
Director of Intensive Care
The Royal Hospitals NHS Trust
London

CASE HISTORY

A 56-year-old man with chronic nephrolithiasis and recurrent urinary tract infections underwent nephrolithotomy. A few hours after returning to the ward he was reviewed by the surgical registrar who noted that he was febrile (38°C), tachycardic (100/min), and tachypnoeic (30 breaths/min), with a poor urine output. The patient also appeared to be confused. Blood and urine were sent for microscopy, culture, and sensitivities, and antibiotics (gentamicin and ampicillin) were given intravenously. Two hours later the patient became hypotensive and was referred to the intensive care team.

EXAMINATION FINDINGS

Temperature 39°C; heart rate 110/min; BP 70/40 mmHg; respiratory rate 35/min. The patients hands were warm and pink with rapid capillary refill and the pulse was 'bounding'.

INVESTIGATIONS

Hb	10.5 gms/dl
WCC	$20,000 \times 10^9$
Platelets	$70\,000 \times 10^9$

Biochemistry		Arterial blood gases	
Sodium	135 mmol/l	pH	7.26
Potassium	4.7 mmol/l	PaO_2	8.2 (breathing room air)
Chloride	100 mmol/l	$PaCO_2$	5.3 kPa
Urea	15 mmol/l	HCO_3	18 mmol/l
Creatinine	150 μmol/l	BE	−6mmol/l

WHAT WAS THE DIAGNOSIS WHEN THE PATIENT WAS FIRST SEEN BY THE SURGICAL REGISTRAR?

The diagnosis was severe sepsis. The patient manifested the features of the systemic inflammatory response syndrome which is defined by the presence of two or more of the following:

(1) temperature $> 38°C$ or $< 36°C$;
(2) heart rate > 90 beats/min.;
(3) respiratory rate > 20 breaths/min or $PaCO_2 < 4.3$ kPa;
(4) white cell count $> 12 \times 10^9$, $< 4 \times 10^9$, or $> 10\%$ immature forms.

In this case there was an obvious source of infection later confirmed microbiologically, allowing the diagnosis of sepsis to be made. When first seen, the patient exhibited signs of hypoperfusion and organ dysfunction (acute alteration in mental state and oliguria) and was therefore by definition, suffering from severe sepsis, a condition which frequently progresses to septic shock/adult respiratory distress syndrome and which is associated with a significant mortality. Investigations performed at this time confirmed the severity of the patient's condition (thrombocytopaenia indicative of disseminated intravascular coagulation (DIC), metabolic acidosis indicative of tissue hypoxia, elevated urea and creatinine, hypoxia, and hyperglycaemia).

WHAT IMMEDIATE MEASURES SHOULD BE INSTITUTED BY THE INTENSIVE CARE TEAM?

(1) ensure the airway is patent and administer oxygen via a face mask;
(2) establish peripheral venous access and expand the circulating volume with a colloid solution;
(3) administer analgesia (small doses of opiates i.v.) as indicated;
(4) appropriate antibiotics have already been given (indeed the consequent bacterial lysis may have been responsible for the patient's deterioration), but the antimicrobial regime may need to be modified later in the light of culture and sensitivity results.

THE PATIENT REMAINS HYPOTENSIVE (90/40 MMHG WITH A PREMORBID BLOOD PRESSURE 130/80 MMHG) AND CAN THEREFORE BE CONSIDERED TO BE SUFFERING FROM SEPTIC SHOCK. HE IS BECOMING MORE CONFUSED AND VERY BREATHLESS. WHAT FURTHER MEASURES WOULD YOU INSTITUTE AT THIS STAGE?

Further measures are:

(1) admit the patient to intensive care;
(2) monitor skin colour, capillary refill time, central and peripheral temperature, the electrocardiogram, and urine flow;
(3) establish central venous and intra-arterial pressure monitoring;
(4) further expand the circulating volume guided by the CVP;
(5) institute mechanical ventilation (early institution of IPPV may improve outcome from septic shock);
(6) the use of 'low-dose' dopamine to improve splanchnic and renal blood flow is controversial and of uncertain value, but many still recommend use of this agent.

FOLLOWING INSTITUTION OF THESE MEASURES THE BP FALLS FURTHER, THE PATIENT REMAINS HYPOXIC, AND THE CHEST X-RAY SHOWS DIFFUSE PULMONARY INFILTRATES. THE BLOOD LACTATE LEVEL IS 5.2 MMOL/L AND THE BASE EXCESS −8 WITH A PH OF 7.22. DISCUSS FURTHER HAEMODYNAMIC MANAGEMENT.

In view of the persistent hypotension combined with a lactic acidosis and oliguria, more aggressive haemodynamic support is clearly indicated. The first priority is to ensure that the circulating volume is adequate. Under these circumstances most would recommend pulmonary artery catheterization and determination of the pulmonary artery occlusion pressure.

Careful monitoring of pulmonary artery and left ventricular filling pressures is particularly important in this patient who has the signs of pulmonary oedema/early adult respiratory distress syndrome.

The optimal filling pressure should be determined by finding the wedge pressure at which left ventricular stroke work index plateaus, although in view of the risk of ARDS lower wedge pressures may be acceptable provided cardiac index and mean arterial measure can be maintained. If the patient remains hypotensive the administration of vasopressor or inotropic agents is indicated. If, as is likely, haemodynamic monitoring confirms that the patient is vasodilated with a high cardiac output, noradrenaline infusion should be used to restore mean arterial pressure to at least 80 mmHg, or to the premorbid value in those with pre-existing hypertension; the systemic vascular resistance index should not be allowed to rise above about 1500 dynes/sec/cm^{-5}. Dobutamine can then be used to achieve an adequate cardiac output but, because it is a potent vasodilator, this agent should in general only be given once the BP has been restored with noradrenaline. Adrenaline is a cheap, and effective, alternative agent for the management of septic shock which, unlike the dobutamine/noradrenaline combination, can be used relatively safely when pulmonary artery catheterization is not possible.

The efficacy of haemodynamic support can be assessed by monitoring serial blood lactate levels. Falling lactate levels, with resolution of metabolic acidosis, suggests adequate haemodynamic support, whereas persistently elevated lactate levels are associated with an extremely poor prognosis. Although it has been suggested that elevation of systemic oxygen delivery (DO_2) and oxygen uptake (VO_2) to levels that some have called 'supranormal' might improve outcome in patients with septic shock, it now seems that this is unlikely. Indeed, in some cases aggressive attempts to boost VO_2 may be detrimental. Neither does treatment targeted to a cardiac index of 4.5 l/min/m^2 or a mixed venous oxygen saturation at or above 70% appear to be beneficial. Nevertheless, it may not be unreasonable in selected cases to explore the dynamic relationship between DO_2 and VO_2 once volume resuscitation is complete and BP has been restored, in an attempt to establish whether survivor values can be equalled or exceeded with only moderate inotropic support. If this is the case, the prospects for survival are good. In those who fail to respond to, or who become refactory to noradrenaline, angiotensin may prove effective. The use of nitric oxide synthase inhibitors remains experimental.

Conventionally, extreme acidosis is said to depress myocardial contractility and may limit the response to vasopressor agents. Attempts to correct acidosis with intravenous bicarbonate may, however, be detrimental. Additional carbon dioxide is generated and because carbon dioxide, but not the bicarbonate ion, readily diffuses across the cell membrane, intracellular pH is further reduced. Other dangers include sodium overload, hyperosmolality and a left shift of the oxyhaemoglobin dissociation curve. Also ionized calcium levels may be reduced and, in combination with the fall in intracellular pH, may be responsible for impaired myocardial performance. Experimental and clinical studies do not support the administration of intravenous sodium bicarbonate to patients with lactic acidosis and treatment should concentrate on correcting the cause, while acidosis is most safely controlled by hyperventilation.

IN VIEW OF THE SEVERITY OF THIS PATIENT'S CONDITION, SHOULD ADJUNCTIVE THERAPY BE CONSIDERED?

Because many of the manifestations of sepsis/septic shock, including the haemodynamic changes and vital organ damage, are mediated by an uncontrolled dissemination of the inflammatory response, it has been postulated that mortality might be reduced by inhibiting the mediators of this response. To date, this approach has, however, been generally disappointing. Although for many years high dose corticosteroids were widely used in the management of shock, well-designed clinical trials eventually demonstrated that large doses of methylprednisolone do not improve outcome in severe sepsis or septic shock, even when administered within a few hours of the diagnosis. Similarly, the use of non-steroidal anti-inflammatory agents, prostacyclin, opiate antagonists and monoclonal antibodies directed against endotoxin, various cytokines or their receptors cannot at present be recommended for general use in the management of sepsis/septic shock.

Currently, there is considerable interest in the potential of naturally occurring cytokine antagonists, soluble receptors and receptor antagonists, as well as bactericidal permeability increasing protein and N-acetylcysteine, amongst many others.

The importance of surgical drainage or removal of the source of infection when possible cannot be overemphasized.

KEY POINTS

1. Early recognition of sepsis and severe sepsis, combined with prompt intervention, may prevent deterioration to multiple organ failure and improve outcome. Delays in treatment are likely to be associated with the development of refractory tissue hypoxia.
2. Adequate volume replacement, restoration of BP to premorbid levels, and maintenance of a cardiac output within the normal range are essential. In those with established septic shock, this usually requires haemodynamic monitoring with a pulmonary artery catheter.
3. Targeting of 'supranormal' values for CI, DO_2, and VO_2 is not recommended.
4. Adjunctive therapies are, at present, of unproven value.
5. When possible, surgical drainage or removal of the source of infection is essential.

FURTHER READING

Hinds, C. and Watson, D. (1995) Manipulating hemodynamics and oxygen transport in critically ill patients. *N.Engl.J.Med.*, **333**, 1074–5.

Members of the American College of Chest Physicians/Society of Critical Care Medicine Consensus Conference Committee. (1992) Definitions for sepsis and organ failure and guidelines for the use of innovative therapies in sepsis. *Crit.Care Med.* 20, 864–74.

Parrillo, J. E. (1993) Pathogenetic mechanisms of septic shock. *N.Eng.J.Med.*, 328, 1471–7.

4.8 TOXIC SHOCK SYNDROME

B. D. SHARPE FANZCA

Consultant Anaesthetist
Chelsea and Westminster Hospital
London

CASE HISTORY

A 17-year-old girl presented to a district hospital with a 2-day history of mild fever and abdominal discomfort. Examination revealed a rise in temperature to 37.8°C; mildly tender abdomen; and a WCC of 12 000 × 10^9/l. She was transferred to theatre for appendicectomy and 5 minutes post-induction had a cardiac arrest in ventricular fibrillation which was successfully treated with 1 mg of adrenaline and a 200 J shock.

One and a half hours post-arrest the patient was in transit to a tertiary referral centre by helicopter, ventilated, sedated, and paralysed. During the flight, two further episodes of ventricular fibrillation occurred, both responding to defibrillation.

On arrival, BP was 70/50 mmHg. The patient was flushed with no focal signs of disease. Being sedated and paralysed, it was not possible to assess her neurological state. She had a sinus tachycardia of 120/min. and ventricular ectopics. She was warm peripherally and appeared normovolaemic. She was catheterized and a lightly blood-stained tampon was removed.

INVESTIGATIONS

Hb	12.3 gm/dl
WCC	12 000 × 10^9/l
Platelets	223 × 10^9/l

Biochemistry

Sodium	142 mmol/l
Potassium	4.9 mmol/l
Urea	4.7 mmol/l
Creatinine	124 μmol/l

Arterial blood gases (FiO$_2$ 0.5)

PaO$_2$	31 kPa
PaCO$_2$	4.7 kPa

pH   7.29
BE   −5 mmol/l
HCO$_3$ 19 mmol/l

A pulmonary artery catheter was inserted.

Haemodynamic parameters

Mean arterial pressure   60 mmHg
CVP   6 mmHg
Pulmonary artery pressure   25/12 mmHg
PAOP   8 mmHg
Cardiac output   4.5 l/min
SVR   960 dynes/sec/cm^{-5}
PVR   178 dynes/sec/cm^{-5}

WHAT IS THE DIFFERENTIAL DIAGNOSIS? DESCRIBE YOUR MANAGEMENT

With the time course described by this case in an apparently fit girl with a mild illness, an event related to the anaesthetic seemed most likely. A discussion of the events around induction is vital. Particular points of interest are those relating to airway management and endotracheal tube insertion, drugs given intentionally or unintentionally, and adverse reactions. In fact, none of these were applicable in this case. In view of the surgical admission diagnosis the patient was transferred to theatre to perform a laparotomy. She arrested again as she was lifted over to the operating table but could not be resuscitated. Subsequently it was realized that she had toxic shock syndrome.

KEY POINTS

1. In the presence of near normal cardiovascular and biochemical parameters in a young person, the cause of life threatening dysrhythmias is most likely to be found in the area of toxicology.
2. A controversial aspect of management is the recourse to surgical intervention in a patient that demonstrably had unstable cardiac function. It is unlikely that a surgical cause could have created this clinical picture. For instance, if the initial assessment of appendicitis had been indicative of bowel disease then even the evolution of dead bowel might have been expected to have been accompanied with more profound biochemical and cardiovascular disturbance. A surgical approach here was perhaps more an act of despair rather than diagnostic or curative. Reassessment of all patients and critical analysis of previously-made diagnoses is pivotal to good intensive care management.
3. Whilst the presence of a tampon here was a substantial clue to the cause of disease, its absence would not have significantly changed the weighting in favour of a diagnosis of toxic shock syndrome.

FURTHER READING

Freedman, J. D. and Beer, D. J. (1991) Expanding perspectives on the toxic shock syndrome. *Adv.Intern Med.*, **36**, 363–97.

NOTES

Part 5 Neurological disorder

5.1 HEAD INJURY

P. S. WITHINGTON FRCA
Director of Intensive Care
The Royal London Hospital
London

CASE HISTORY

A previously fit, 22-year-old man was admitted to the intensive care unit following a road traffic accident. On arrival at A&E he was in a coma (GCS of 6) and was noted to have a head injury and fractured pelvis. A head CT scan revealed diffuse brain swelling with no focal lesion. Intracranial pressure (ICP) monitoring was instituted and external fixation applied to stabilize the pelvic fractures. Treatment included mannitol 100 g, gelofusine 2 litres, anaesthesia, and ventilation. Midazolam, fentanyl, and pancuronium were used for sedation and muscle relaxation.

INVESTIGATIONS

BP	100/60 mmHg
CVP	3 mmHg
heart rate	132/min
core temperature	38.5°C.
Hb	7.2 g/dl
Intracranial pressure (ICP)	25 mmHg
Blood sugar	15.4 mmol/l

Arterial blood gases (FiO$_2$ 0.4)

PaO$_2$	8 kPa
PaCO$_2$	2.8 kPa
pH	7.45

DISCUSS MANAGEMENT AND TREATMENT

The main aim of treatment after severe head injury is to reduce the amount of secondary cerebral damage caused by ischaemia.

Sedation and ventilation should be maintained until the brain swelling has been controlled.

Immediate management. The arterial PO_2 and hence oxygen saturation, is low. This will reduce the oxygen delivery to the brain. The FiO_2 should be increased and PEEP added if necessary.

Cerebral perfusion pressure (CPP) should be assessed with reference to the mean arterial pressure (MAP) and intracranial pressure (CPP = MAP − ICP). MAP = 73 mmHg, ICP = 25 mmHg, therefore CPP = 48 mmHg. This is too low. In normal subjects cerebral blood flow (CBF) is autoregulated so that it remains fairly constant over a wide range of arterial blood pressure. However, following head injury, autoregulation is impaired and once the CPP falls below 70 mmHg the CBF will fall resulting in cerebral hypoperfusion. CPP should be maintained over 70 mmHg at all times. The quickest way to improve CPP is to raise the BP.

The patient is hypovolaemic, hypotensive, and anaemic. He should receive a rapid blood transfusion; this should raise the BP and so restore CPP to adequate levels. If vigorous fluid therapy fails to produce an adequate BP then a vasopressor such as noradrenaline should be given. Hb should be maintained over 12 g/dl.

Raised ICP *per se* is harmful and should therefore be reduced. With diffuse brain swelling carbon dioxide reactivity is usually well preserved and so hyperventilation may be a useful therapy to reduce ICP. However, excessive hyperventilation can produce cerebral ischaemia by profound vasoconstriction; without extensive monitoring of cerebral oxygenation moderate hyperventilation only ($PaCO_2$ 3.5–4.5 kPa) should be employed. Regular mannitol (500 mg/kg, 8-hourly) decreases ICP, though the exact mechanisms of action are unknown. This treatment should be stopped when the plasma osmolality reaches 320 mosm/l.

Pyrexia is common with autonomic dysfunction following head injury. This increases cerebral oxygen demands ($CMRO_2$) at a time when oxygen supply is decreased. There is increasing evidence that moderate hypothermia (33–35°C) is beneficial in reducing $CMRO_2$ and ICP.

Hyperglycaemia should be avoided. Under anaerobic conditions, glucose metabolism leads to lactic acid formation. This exacerbates intracerebral acidosis and makes ICP more difficult to control. An insulin infusion should be administered to maintain blood glucose in the normal range.

KEY POINTS

1. The most important aspect of head injury management is to reduce secondary brain damage.
2. The mechanisms of damage are complex and ill-understood; however, cerebral ischaemia appears to play a major role.
3. Adequate cerebral perfusion with well-oxygenated blood must be maintained at all times. Repeated brief periods of cerebral hypoperfusion (e.g. while in theatres or CT scan) have an additive detrimental effect on outcome.

FURTHER READING

Jones, P. A., Andrews, P. J. D. Midgley, S., *et al.* (1994) Measuring the burden of secondary insults in head-injured patients during intensive care. *J.Neurosurg.Anaesth.* 6, 4–14.

Miller, J. D., Jones, P. A., Dearden, N. M. and Tocher, J. L. (1992) Progress in the management of head injury. *Br.J.Surg.*, 79, 60–4.

Okada, K. and Okawa, K. (1994) Trauma anaesthesia for central nervous system injuries. *Curr.Opin.Anesth.*, 7, 205–12.

NOTES

5.2 THE POST-OPERATIVE NEUROSURGICAL CASE

M. SMITH FRCA
Consultant Neuroanaesthetist
The National Hospital for Neurology and Neurosurgery
London

CASE HISTORY

A 25-year-old male was admitted with a head injury following a road traffic accident. At the accident site his GCS was 3 and he was intubated and ventilated for transfer. CT scan revealed an acute left-sided extradural haematoma and small frontal lobe contusions. There were no other injuries. The extradural haematoma was evacuated and postoperatively the patient was sedated and ventilated on the intensive care unit. ICP was 12 mmHg. Twelve hours postoperatively his ICP rose to over 30 mmHg and, despite treatment, his left pupil suddenly dilated.

WHAT ARE THE POSSIBLE REASONS FOR HIS SUDDEN DETERIORATION?

A postoperative neurosurgical patient may deteriorate because of bleeding or brain swelling and either could be the cause in this patient. Re-accumulation of the extradural haematoma, post-surgical bleeding or cerebral oedema (secondary to the extradural haematoma or the frontal contusions) can all occur within the first few postoperative hours. Finally, occult intracerebral haemorrhages may present some hours after closed head injury and may be associated with a sudden rise in ICP and localizing signs.

An urgent CT scan must be carried out to confirm the diagnosis. Unexplained rises in ICP, changes in conscious level (in unsedated patients), and new localizing neurological signs all require urgent CT scanning.

DISCUSS THE MANAGEMENT OF THE PATIENT WITH PARTICULAR REFERENCE TO THE TREATMENT OF RAISED INTRACRANIAL PRESSURE AND THE PROBLEMS OF SUCH THERAPY.

In the absence of a surgically treatable lesion, intracranial hypertension may be managed by control of intracranial blood volume, by use of osmotic agents, or by manipulation of cerebral metabolic factors. Slight head up tilt (15–20°C) and moderate neck flexion allow optimal cerebral venous drainage and reduction in ICP but may be accompanied by a fall in systemic blood pressure which may compromise CPP. Moderate hyperventilation ($PaCO_2$ 3.8–4.2 kPa) has been the cornerstone of treatment of intracranial hypertension for many years. It is accepted that the fall in ICP occurs secondary to cerebral vasoconstriction and a fall in cerebral blood volume. Other advantages of hyperventilation include reversal of CSF acidosis and restoration of cerebral autoregulation. Overzealous hyperventilation may, however, provoke a dangerous decrease in CBF and precipitate cerebral ischaemia. Indomethacin and dihydroergotamine also cause falls in ICP secondary to constriction of cerebral vessels.

Mannitol lowers ICP when used as a single dose on demand, improves blood rheology, and is a free radical scavenger. Chronic mannitol therapy may, however, lead to hypernatraemia and hyperosmolality. Reduction in cerebral metabolic rate ($CMRO_2$) is accompanied by a fall in CBF and ICP. Small decreases in temperature have been used to control ICP and there has recently been renewed interest in this technique. Barbiturates increase cerebrovascular resistance and reduce ICP through metabolic suppression of oxygen consumption. Falls in BP may compromise CPP. Chronic use of barbiturates is associated with other problems due to accumulation of the drug and has never been shown to improve outcome.

More recently, propofol has been used to reduce $CMRO_2$ and ICP in neurosurgical patients. During propofol infusion, CPP can be supported by adequate cardiovascular filling. Meanwhile the carbon dioxide reactivity of cerebral vessels is maintained with advantages for the concurrent use of hyperventilation. Propofol sedation can readily be deepened prior to invasive interventions and lightened for neurological assessment.

WHAT OTHER TECHNIQUES MAY BE HELPFUL FOR MONITORING CEREBRAL FUNCTION IN THIS PATIENT?

Measurement of ICP is helpful in guiding therapy in brain injured patients but gives no indication of the cerebral metabolic state. Placement of a jugular bulb catheter allows continuous monitoring of jugular bulb oxygen saturation ($SjvO_2$) and intermittent measurement of cerebral venous lactate levels. The normal values for $SjvO_2$ lie between 55–75%. Levels of 45–55% reflect a reduction in CBF and an increase in cerebral oxygen extraction whereas levels < 45% may indicate global ischamia. High $SjvO_2$ values (> 75%) may occur because of cerebral hyperaemia. Other patient variables as well as incorrect catheter placement may affect values of $SjvO_2$, and trends rather than absolute values, interpreted in relation to the clinical state of the patient, are more helpful than isolated readings. The lactate oxygen index (LOI) has recently been used to assess the relative amounts of anaerobic and aerobic cerebral metabolism. The LOI is calculated by the ratio of the arteriovenous lactate difference to arteriovenous oxygen content difference. The normal value is < 0.03. It has been suggested that $SjvO_2$ < 55% with a LOI of > 0.08 may indicate cerebral ischaemia.

KEY POINTS

1. In the postoperative neurosurgical patient, changes in conscious level, unexplained rises in ICP, and new localizing neurological signs must be investigated by urgent CT to exclude a surgically treatable problem.
2. Moderate hyperventilation (3.8–4.2 kPa) has long been the cornerstone of the treatment of intracranial hypertension but has never been shown to improve outcome. Overzealous hyperventilation may precipitate cerebral ischaemia if CBF falls below a critical level.
3. ICP monitoring is helpful in guiding therapy after acute brain injury but provides no information about the metabolic state of the brain. A jugular bulb catheter allows continuous jugular venous oximetry, as well as measurement of cerebral venous lactate levels, which give indirect assessments of cerebral metabolism.

FURTHER READING

Dearden, N. M. (1991) Jugular bulb venous oxygen saturation in the management of severe head injury. *Curr.Opin.Anaesth.*, 4, 279–86.

Lewis, S. B., Reilly, P. L., and Myburgh, J. A. (1994) Developments in intracranial pressure monitoring and investigaion of head-injured patients. In (ed. G. J. Dobb, J. Bion, H. Burchardi, R. P. Dellinger) *Current topics in intensive care.* W. B. Saunders Company, London.

Smith, M. (1994) Postoperative neurosurgical care. *Curr. Anaesth. Crit. Care,* 5, 29–35.

5.3 GUILLAIN–BARRÉ SYNDROME

N. HIRSCH FRCA
Consultant Anaesthetist, The Batten Harris Intensive Care Unit
The National Hospital for Neurology and Neurosurgery
London

CASE HISTORY

A 70 kg, 55-year-old man was admitted to A&E with a 24-hour history of increasing shortness of breath and difficulty in swallowing. One week previously he suffered an upper respiratory tract infection, followed by pain and paraesthesiae in both feet and weakness in both legs, making it difficult for him to walk without help.

EXAMINATION FINDINGS

The patient was noted to be tachypnoeic, using accessary respiratory muscles, and exhausted. He was hypertensive (BP 200/120 mmHg) with a tachycardia (120/min). Lung fields were clear to auscultation although both bases had poor air entry. There was paradoxical abdominal movement on inspiration and his cough was bovine in nature. Abdominal examination revealed a distended bladder. Neurological examination revealed normal intellectual function. Cranial nerve examination showed bilateral facial weakness, partial ophthalmoplegia, and reduced tongue and palatal movement with pooling of saliva in the pyriform fossae. Distal and proximal muscle weakness was found in all limbs but the legs were more severely affected than the arms. Tendon reflexes were absent at the knees and ankles and were reduced in the arms. Examination of the sensory system revealed no abnormality apart from mild proprioceptive loss.

INVESTIGATIONS

Vital capacity (VC), measured using a facemask, was 900ml. Arterial blood gas analysis revealed:

PaO_2	8.4 kPa
$PaCO_2$	9.0kPa
pH	7.31
HCO_3	32 mmol/l

DISCUSS MANAGEMENT AND TREATMENT

Examination of the respiratory system revealed paradoxical abdominal movement on inspiration, indicating severe diaphragmatic weakness; this was supported by the finding of a low vital capacity (normal 65 ml/kg). Arterial blood gas analysis confirmed type 2 respiratory failure. Neurological examination revealed poor bulbar function with inadequate swallowing of saliva. The patient was therefore intubated, both to support ventilation and to protect the airway from aspiration. A nasotracheal tube was inserted as was a nasogastric tube. A urinary catheter was passed. The patient was sedated for the first 24 hours of ventilation.

Although there are a number of causes of a generalized motor paralysis (e.g. myasthenia gravis, botulism, poliomyelitis, periodic paralysis, porphyria), the most common cause is Guillain–Barré syndrome (GBS). The history and clinical features of this patient are typical of this condition.

Apart from a careful history and examination, confirmation of the diagnosis of the condition requires examination of the cerebrospinal fluid and electromyography. In this case, cerebrospinal fluid examination revealed a protein of 0.93 g/l (normal < 0.5 g/l), two white cells, and a normal glucose. Electromyographic studies revealed marked slowing of nerve conduction with increases in distal motor latencies. No axonal loss was demonstrated.

Treatment of GBS falls into two categories – supportive and specific. Supportive treatment requires meticulous nursing and medical care, including regular chest and limb physiotherapy, frequent turning of the patient, enteral (and rarely parenteral) feeding, treatment of pain, and prophylaxis against deep vein thrombosis. Autonomic features are common and were seen in this case, with tachycardia and hypertension persisting despite sedation. They responded to propanolol 5 mg twice a day, and intermittent nifedipine.

Specific treatment of GBS consists of plasma exchange or the administration of human normal immunoglobulin (lglv). Plasma exchange speeds recovery if performed within two weeks of the onset of neurological symptoms. If plasma exchange is contraindicated due to infection or haemodynamic instability, lglv should be given. Initial trials are encouraging and lglv is superceding plasma exchange as primary treatment for GBS in many centres. Corticosteroids have no role.

Despite exchange, the patient's vital capacity fell to a nadir of 200 ml and tracheostomy was performed. Three weeks after the initiation of ventilation, vital capacity (VC) started to rise and after a further 2 weeks he was successfully weaned from mechanical ventilation. After removal of his tracheostomy he was discharged from ITU for rehabilitation, following which he made a complete recovery.

KEY POINTS

1. GBS is the most common cause of a rapidly progressing weakness. Approximately 30% of patients require mechanical ventilation.
2. A raised CSF protein (especially after the first week), in the presence of a normal cell count and EMG studies demonstrating demyelination, help confirm the diagnosis.
3. Recovery is accelerated if plasma exchange is performed within 2 weeks of the onset of neurological symptoms. Recent work suggests intravenous normal immunoglobulin is as effective as exchange.

FURTHER READING

Guillain–Barré syndrome study group. (1985) Plasmapheresis and acute Guillain–Barré syndrome. *Neurology*, 35, 1096–1104.

Ng, K. K. P., Howard, R. S., Fish, D. R., Hirsch, N. P., Wiles, C. M., Murray, N. M. F., *et al.* (1995) Management and outcome of severe Guillain–Barré syndrome. *Q J Med.*, 88, 234–50.

Van der Meche, F. G. A., Schmitz, P. I. M., and the Dutch Guillain–Barré study group. (1992) A randomized trial comparing intravenous immunoglobulin and plasma exchange in Guillain-Barré syndrome. *N.Engl.J.Med.*, 326, 1123–9.

NOTES

5.4 CRITICAL CARE NEUROPATHY

J. H. COAKLEY FRCP
Consultant Physician
Intensive Care Unit
St Bartholomew's Hospital
London

CASE HISTORY

A 68-year-old, previously fit woman was admitted to the ITU following a respiratory arrest. After resuscitation and investigation she was found to have septic shock due to pneumonia. Her initial management was complicated by the development of a pneumothorax, requiring intercostal drain insertion. After blood, sputum, and urine cultures were taken she was treated with intravenous cefuroxime and erythromycin. Subsequently, pneumococcal septicaemia was confirmed.

During the subsequent course of her ITU stay she suffered acute respiratory distress syndrome, requiring 100% oxygen, sedation, and muscle relaxants to overcome high lung inflation pressures. Cardiovascular failure necessitated insertion of a pulmonary artery flotation catheter for optimization of vasoactive drug therapy, leading to treatment with noradrenaline. Despite adequate resuscitation, acute tubular necrosis developed and she required continuous veno-venous haemodiafiltration. Intestinal failure led to 2 weeks total parental nutrition.

After 4 weeks of mechanical ventilation the lung lesions had resolved, but not the renal failure. Sedative drugs were discontinued with a view to weaning from mechanical ventilation and extubating the patient's trachea. Twenty-four hours later the patient was able to open her eyes to command, but was otherwise immobile and unresponsive. The limbs were flaccid and areflexic, and sensation clinically unimpaired but difficult to assess.

WHAT IS THE DIAGNOSIS?

Almost certainly the critical illness neuropathy (CIN), a common accompaniment of prolonged intensive care. Early reports suggested that this only occurred in sepsis and multiple organ failure, but it is becoming increasingly recognized after prolonged ITU stay, whether or not associated with these factors. Its aetiology is unknown, and there is no clear evidence of a relationship to the use of neuromuscular blocking agents. It is possible that the condition could be Guillain–Barré syndrome (GBS), which may complicate such severe illnesses. The patient may also have suffered necrotizing muscle breakdown, which may occur in sepsis and multiple organ failure, particularly renal failure, but this is not usually associated with areflexia.

WHAT TWO INVESTIGATIONS ARE NECESSARY TO CONFIRM IT?

Neurophysiological studies; not just nerve conduction velocities which are almost invariably normal in CIN. In demyelination, nerve conduction is usually slowed but the findings in axonal neuropathies differ. Stimulation of the nerves in axonal loss leads to a reduction in the amplitude of the transmitted signal rather than a slowing of the signal. This is due to loss of conducting tissue in the axons; hence there is usually a reduction in compound muscle action potentials and sensory action potentials. There is often evidence of denervation, such as spontaneous muscle fibrillation on electromyography.

GBS is usually associated with reduced nerve conduction velocities because of demyelination. Necrotising myopathy is associated with myopathic changes in the electromyogram.

Lumbar puncture and cerebrospinal fluid (CSF) examination should be carried out to exclude GBS. The CSF in CIN is normal, but in GBS contains increased protein with no cells.

WHAT IS THE TREATMENT?

There is no specific therapy. The patient's respiratory system should be supported, and weaning will almost certainly be prolonged. It is imperative that such patients are not assumed to have irreversible ventilator dependence, and that weaning is allowed to progress at its own pace rather than that of the attendant medical staff. Once the patient can breathe spontaneously, rehabilitation will be necessary to facilitate mobilization and self-caring.

FURTHER READING

Coakley, J. H., Edwards, R. H. T., McClelland, P., Bone, J. M. and Helliwell, T. R. (1990) Occult skeletal muscle necrosis associated with renal failure. *Br.Med.J.*, **301**, 370

Coakley, J. H., Nagendran, K., Honavar, M., and Hinds, C. J. (1993) Preliminary observations on the neuromuscular abnormalities in patients with organ failure and sepsis. *Intensive Care Med.*, **19**, 323–8.

Coakley, J. H., Nagendran, K., Ormerod, I. E. C., Ferguson, C. and Hinds, C. J. (1992) Prolonged neurogenic weakness in patients requiring mechanical ventilation for acute airflow limitation. *Chest*, **5**, 1413–16.

Helliwell, T. R., Coakley, J. H., Wagenmakers, A. J. M., *et al.* (1991) Necrotising myopathy in critically ill patients. *J.Path.*, **164**, 307–14.

NOTES

7.4 PHAEOCHROMOCYTOMA

G. BELLINGAN MRCP
Lecturer and Honorary Senior Registrar
Intensive Care Unit
Middlesex Hospital
UCL
London

CASE HISTORY

A 29-year-old male was admitted with a 6-hour history of nausea, vomiting, and abdominal pain.

On examination he was pyrexial and sweating with a heart rate of 70/min and BP of 155/85 mmHg. There was mild epigastric tenderness only. Apart from a white cell count of 18×10^9/l, his admission haematology, biochemistry, and microbiology tests were entirely normal as was his chest X-ray and ECG. The next morning he developed acute pulmonary oedema requiring mechanical ventilation. He suffered two asystolic arrests and was eventually stabilized on an adrenaline infusion. His chest X-ray was consistent with pulmonary oedema; PAOP was 24 mmHg; and cardiac output was 5.5 l/min. His ECG remained normal and there was no rise in his cardiac enzymes. An echocardiogram demonstrated mild ventricular hypokinesia and abdominal ultrasound showed a 6 cm mass over the right kidney.

He deteriorated further with a falling cardiac output and rising wedge pressure which was briefly stabilized by plasma exchange, but after 2 days he died. Post-mortem demonstrated a phaeochromocytoma.

DISCUSS THE DIAGNOSIS OF HIS CONDITION

Phaeochromocytoma is not always an easy diagnosis to make and, as this case demonstrates, it does not always present with a hypertensive crisis. A recent review of 62 deaths from phaeochromocytoma in the UK by a post-mortem survey revealed that typical symptoms (palpitations, episodic sweating, dyspnoea, and headache) were present for 3 months in only 60% of cases, with little difference between benign or malignant disease. Bone pain was the only symptom that distinguished benign (absent in all cases) from malignant disease (present in 20%). Thirty per cent of deaths from phaeochromocytoma in this series had had only a short preceding history; all of these presented with vomiting, most with acute abdominal pain, and over 80% had acute dyspnoea from left ventricular failure, although other prospective studies suggest a lower incidence of abdominal pain. Physical findings were non-specific, 70% being hypertensive but 10% hypotensive, and 50% had signs of heart failure. An abdominal mass was palpable in only 13%. Although a family history is useful, this was present in only a minority of cases.

INVESTIGATIONS

Elevated white cell counts are common and non-specific, urinalysis is unhelpful, and urinary vanillyl mandelic acid (VMA) can be misleading as in 25% of cases this is normal. In patients on inotropes, VMA measurement is meaningless. Furthermore, the stress of hospital admission often elevates catecholamine levels abnormally. This test is also very slow, taking usually more than 48 hours between collection and result. Urinary metanephrine levels may be more specific but will be just as slow.

Abdominal ultrasound has a 60% specificity; CT is better and t2 weighted magnetic resonance imaging can clearly demonstrate a phaeochromocytoma due to the density of the chromaffin cells. A benign suprarenal mass is not an uncommon finding but the likelihood of it being a phaeochromocytoma is strong if it is more than 4 cm. However, many phaeochromocytomas are significantly smaller than this. I^{131} meta-iodobenzylguanidine (MIBG) scans, although very sensitive, suffer from the problem of being slow, again with a delay of more than 24 hours between injection and first result. Thus, not only is there a problem in suspecting the diagnosis from the non-specific signs and symptoms but there is difficulty in confirming it.

TREATMENT

Plasma exchange was used as a last ditch attempt to improve left ventricular function in the absence of a clear diagnosis. The rationale for its use was to attempt to remove putative myocardial depressant factors that might have contributed to the cardiac failure. It did, in fact, seem to stabilize the situation briefly. Other desperate measures might have included the use of an intra-aortic balloon pump or extra corporeal membrane oxygenation. Although most people would use such techniques in young patients *in extremis*, and there are anecdotal reports of benefit, there are no good controlled trials suggesting their use routinely. In this case, the hope was that sufficient stability could be restored to allow further investigation and treatment of the adrenal mass.

KEY POINTS

1. One should have a high index of suspicion of phaeochromocytoma with any unexplained case of pulmonary oedema, especially when there is vomiting and abdominal pain.
2. Phaeochromocytoma presenting with heart failure or abdominal pain is often only diagnosed at autopsy.
3. The investigations of choice are an ultrasound scan, and if that is negative a CT or MRI scan. Any mass of 4 cm or more is likely to be pathological and surgery should be contemplated immediately if the patient is very unwell.

FURTHER READING

Gan, T. G., Miller, R. F., Webb, A. R., and Russell, R. C. (1994) Phaeochromocytoma presenting as acute hyperamylasaemia and multi-organ failure. *Can.J.Anaesth.*, **41**, 244–7.

Platts, J. K., Drew, P. J. T. and Harvey, J. N. (1995) Death from phaeochromocytoma: lessons from a post-mortem survey. *J.Roy.Coll.Phys. London*, **29**, 299–306.

Ross, E. J. and Griffith, E. D. W. (1989) The clinical presentation of phaeochromocytoma. *Q.J.Med.*, **71**, 485–96.

Sardesai, S. H., Mourant, A. J., Sivathandon, Y., Farrow, R. and Gibbons, D. O. (1990) Phaeochromocytoma and catecholamine-induced cardiomyopathy presenting as heart failure. *Br. Heart J.* **63**, 234–7.

Spencer, E., Pycock, C. and Lytle, J. P. (1993) Phaeochromocytoma presenting as acute circulatory collapse and abdominal pain. *Int. Care Med.*, **19**, 356–7.

St. John Sutton, M. G., Sheps, S. G., Lie, J. T. (1991) Prevalence of clinically unsuspected phaeochromocytoma. Review of a 50 year autopsy series. *Clin.Proc.* **56**, 354–60.

NOTES

A. J. Ellis MRCP
Senior Registrar in Hepatology
and
J. A. Wendon MRCP
Senior Lecturer and Honorary Consultant in Hepatology
Institute of Liver Studies Kings College Hospital
Kings College Hospital
London

CASE HISTORY

A 35-year-old lady was found collapsed and disorientated on the floor of her flat. She had previously complained to her partner of abdominal pain, nausea, and vomiting for 24 hours.

In casualty a medical history revealed mild asthma, alcohol consumption of 20–30 units per week, and no recreational drug use.

EXAMINATION FINDINGS

On examination her GCS was 12, muscle tone was normal, and there was no neck stiffness. The respiratory rate was 30/min; pulse 120/minute; and BP 90/40 mmHg. The abdomen was soft, there was no organomegaly, and no evidence of jaundice.

INVESTIGATIONS

Biochemistry

Sodium	135 mmol/l
Potassium	4.0 mmol/l
Urea	2.0 mmol/l
Creatinine	250 μmol/l
Glucose	1.5 mmol/l
Hb	13 g/dl
WCC	15×10^9/l
platelets	70×10^9/l
Total protein	70 g/l

Albumin   43 g/l
Bilirubin   55 μmol/l
AST   > 10 000 iu/l
Calcium   2.40 mmol/l
Phosphate   0.46 mmol/l
INR   5.5
APPT   40 secs (normal 35)
FDP   < 0.25 mg/dl
CT scan of head: normal
Paracetamol level   45 mmol/l
Salicylate undetectable

Arterial blood gases

pH   7.28
PaCO$_2$ 2.5 kPa
PaO$_2$ 15 kPa
HCO$_3$ 14 mmol/l

WHAT IS THE DIAGNOSIS AND DESCRIBE YOUR MANAGEMENT

A diagnosis of paracetomol toxicity and acute liver failure (ALF) was made, and 50% dextrose given intravenously, with prompt improvement of conscious level. A specialized liver unit offering transplant services was contacted who agreed to take the patient (see Table 1). Over several hours, the patient again became drowsy, interspersed with aggressive behaviour – features compatible with grade 3 encephalopathy. Despite colloid loading, the tachycardia persisted with hypotension (BP 100/40 mmHg) The patient was therefore transferred to the ITU where she was electively ventilated, sedated, and paralysed, and an arterial line was placed. During transfer to the liver unit, mean arterial pressure fell and adrenaline was commenced. At the same time she developed a dilated right pupil which responded to mannitol. On arrival, investigations revealed pH 7.15, $PaCO_2$ 2.5 kPa, PaO_2 18 kPa, HCO_3 8 mmol/l, INR 10.5, creatinine 310 μmol/l, and lactate 8 mmol/l. Fulfilling criteria for liver transplantation, she was put on the supraurgent transplant register.

Criteria for referral to King's Liver Unit (Paracetamol toxicity)

Evidence of encephalopathy; a prothrombin time (secs) of more than the number of hours post-overdose; renal failure in the absence of facilities for continuous veno-venous, haemofiltration (CVVHD); and arterial pH of < 7.3.

Criteria for transplantation as used at King's Liver Unit (Paracetamol toxicity)

Arterial pH of < 7.3 following rehydration or all three of the following: (i) grade 3 encephalopathy; (ii) serum creatinine > 300 μmol/l; (iii) prothrombin time > 100 secs.

Table 1   Criteria currently in use to identify patients who should be transferred to a liver unit and those in whom transplantation is urgently required.

Criteria for referral to King's Liver Unit	• evidence of encephalopathy • a prothrombin time (secs) of more than the number of hours post overdose • renal failure in the absence of facilities for CVVHD • arterial pH of <7.3
Criteria for transplantation as used at King's Liver Unit	• arterial pH of <7.3 following rehydration or all of the following • grade III encephalopathy • serum creatinine > 300 umol/l • prothrombin time >100 seconds

Patients should be commenced on N-acetylcysteine (NAC), regardless of the time between overdose and presentation, because of demonstrated benefits to haemodynamics, oxygen utilization, cerebral oedema, and survival.

A central line is inserted and the CVP maintained at between 6–10 cmH$_2$O. Clotting factors are not usually given for this procedure as complications are rare and the INR is important in establishing the need for liver transplantation. Volume repletion with 4.5% human albumin solution up to 3 litres may be required before an adequate CVP can be obtained.

Hypophosphataemia is very common in paracetomol toxicity and patients should be treated with intravenous phosphates, although caution is required in renal impairment.

The benefit of early systemic broadspectrum antibiotics has been established in prospective controlled trials. Oral amphotericin is given as fungal prophylaxis because of infection rates up to 35%.

Prophylaxis against gastric ulceration is with sucralfate unless vomiting is so severe that an intravenous agent (proton pump inhibitor or H$_2$ blocker) is indicated.

In patients who do not develop encephalopathy, blood should be assayed 12-hourly for INR, arterial pH, and serum creatinine. N-acetylcysteine should be continued until the INR falls below 2.

Renal failure may develop in the absence of significant liver damage and should be managed with CVVHD until day 6 post-overdose, as haemodialysis may provoke coma and cerebral oedema during this period.

Once grade 2 encephalopathy develops, further deterioration should be anticipated, particularly with respect to haemodynamic instability and cerebral oedema. Prior to transfer of such patients to a liver unit, the patient should be intubated to protect the airway and adequate vascular access established. An adrenaline infusion should be at hand in addition to mannitol and 50% dextrose. During transfer, pupil reactions should be assessed every 15 minutes and eyelids should not be taped. Blood sugar should be checked on departure and at 15 minute intervals.

All hypotensive patients should be monitored with a pulmonary flotation catheter to enable calculation of haemodynamic variables. CVVHD utilizing either prostacycline or heparin as an anticoagulant is required to support those patients with renal failure. To allow the early recognition and management of cerebral oedema, an extradural intracranial pressure bolt is inserted under FFP cover in those patients proceeding to transplantation.

Note: Indications for transplantation in liver failure not due to paracetamol toxicity are different. See Table 2.

Table 2 General indications for liver transplantation in critically ill patients with acute liver failure. (NB patients should be referred to a liver unit before they reach this stage)

The patient should satisfy three of the following:

- evidence of encephalopathy
- age <10 or >40 years
- non-A, non-B or drug-induced hepatatis
- prothrombin time >50 secs
- serum bilirubin >300 umol/l
- jaundice to encephalopathy time >7 days.

Patients with Wilson's disease, Budd–Chiari syndrome or liver disease in pregnancy should be discussed individually with the liver unit.

KEY POINTS

1. Make early and regular contact with a specialized liver unit.
2. The INR is the most valuable predictor of prognosis and the need for transplantation. Bleeding from line sites is uncommon and clotting factor replacement is not usually required if the platelets are $> 70 \times 10^9/l$.
3. Once grade 2 encephalopathy is present; deterioration is frequently rapid and ventilation is preferable prior to patient transfer.

FURTHER READING

Keays, R., Harrison, P. M., Wendon, J. A., Forbes, A., Grove, C., Alexander, G. J., et al. (1991) Intravenous acetylcysteine in paracetomol-induced fulminant hepatic failure: a prospective controlled trial. *Br.Med.J.*, **303** (6809), 1026–9.

O'Grady, J. G., Alexander, G. J., Hayllar, K. M., and Williams, R. (1989) Early indicators of prognosis in fulminant hepatic failure. *Gastroenterology*, **97** (2), 439–45.

Rolando, N., Harvey, F., Brahm, J., Philpott-Howard, J., Alexander, G., Gimson, A., et al. (1990) Prospective study of bacterial infection in acute liver failure: an analysis of 50 patients. *Hepatology*, **11**(1), 49–53.

NOTES

Part 8 Obstetric and paediatrics

8.1 HAEMOLYSIS, ELEVATED LIVER ENZYMES, AND LOW PLATELETS (HELLP)

G. C. HANSON FRCP FFARCS
Late Consultant Physician
Intensive Care Unit, Whipps Cross Hospital
London

CASE HISTORY

A white female aged 36 years, with two previous pregnancies both complicated by hypertension towards term, was admitted at 28 weeks pregnancy with a 3-day history of malaise, nausea, and epigastric pain.

On admission she had minimal facial and ankle oedema; BP was 160/90 mmHg. There was minimal tenderness in the right hypochondrium. Over the next 3 days the patient deteriorated with increasing oedema, the onset of a headache with irritability, and development of haematuria. She then developed sudden hypotension, tachycardia, and oliguria.

INVESTIGATIONS

Biochemistry

Sodium	130 mmol/l
Potassium	5.6 mmol/l
Urea	7.5 mmol/l
Creatinine	120 μmol/l
Hb	9.0 g/dl
Platelets	80×10^9/l
PT (secs)	12
APTT	30
Serum urate	100 μmol/l
Alkaline phosphatase	500 iu/l
AST	50 iu/l
Bilirubin	30 μmol/l
Urine protein	600 mg/24 hour
Blood film:	burr cells and shistocytes present
CVP at time of collapse:	0 mmHg

DISCUSS DIAGNOSIS AND MANAGEMENT

This patient has the HELLP syndrome (Haemolysis, Elevated Liver enzymes, and Low Platelets) which affects 2–12% of the severe pre-eclamptic population. Typically, the patient is a white, multiparous woman with a history of poor pregnancy outcome. The onset is variable: 70% are antepartum, and 11% < 27 weeks pregnant. Common manifestations are weight gain with generalized oedema. It is important to stress that 30% of patients may have mild hypertension and in 20% the BP is normal without proteinuria.

The presentation may be atypical with malaise, jaundice, evidence of bleeding, or pain in the right hypochondrium. Misdiagnosis is common. At onset, most patients demonstrate thrombocytopenia and evidence of intravascular haemolysis but show no evidence of disseminated intravascular coagulation until the syndrome is severe.

Sibai suggested the following laboratory tests for the diagnosis of the HELLP syndrome:

1) haemolysis – abnormal peripheral film, increased bilirubin, increased lactic dehydrogenase;
2) atypical abnormal liver enzymes;
3) thrombocytopenia – platelets < 100×10^9/l.

The classic hepatitic lesion is periportal or focal parenchymal necrosis and may be complicated by intrahepatic haemorrhage, subcapsular haematoma, and liver rupture. A sudden drop in BP, tachycardia, and a right atrial pressure of zero is consistent with hypovolaemia.

Differential diagnosis. Hypotension may be due to (i) therapy – eg the use of a hypotensive agent or epidural blockade; or (ii) blood loss – abruptio placentae, rupture of an intra-abdominal arterial aneurysm, or ruptured liver. Differentiation can be made by abdominal palpation, ultrasound of the abdomen, evidence of vaginal loss of blood, or blood in the syringe with an intraperitoneal tap.

Blood disorders may be caused by thrombotic thrombocytopenic purpura, haemolytic uraemic syndrome, or HELLP syndrome superimposed upon underlying non-pregnancy-related hypertensive disease.

Management. The only definitive treatment for the patient with the HELLP syndrome is delivery, regardless of gestational age. The maternal mortality in this condition is 0–24% and perinatal mortality 7.7–60%. As many as 44% of the infants are growth retarded. In view of the high maternal mortality, delivery should not be delayed. The mode of delivery depends upon the severity of the condition, the stage of pregnancy, and the favourability of the cervix.

In conjunction with delivery, right atrial pressure monitoring is essential to regulate the circulating blood volume. Control of hypertension should be with the hypotensive parenteral agent of choice, e.g. hydralazine or labetalol. Labetalol is contraindicated where there is bronchospasm and hydralazine is preferable if there is volume overload. Sublingual nifedipine is effective, works within 15 minutes of application, and acts synergistically with the parenteral hypotensive agent. Both can produce a tachycardia. Where the patient is irritable, sedation with diazepam may be considered; however, this may produce foetal sedation and compromise the patient's airway. Magnesium sulphate is now the drug of choice for eclampsia and may be beneficial to the infant. When the patient has convulsed or is irritable and there is concern about airway control, induction, intubation, and general anaesthesia is the preferred option for emergency caesarian section.

Prior to caesarean section it may be necessary to replace clotting factors with FFP and or cryoprecipitate. Platelet infusion should be considered if the platelet count is $< 80 \times 10^9/l$ or falling rapidly. It is essential to monitor urine sodium and potassium, and to observe urine output in order to detect the early onset of acute renal failure. Acute renal failure occurs in around 5% of patients with the syndrome antepartum, and 12% of patients manifesting postpartum.

In the presence of haemolysis, potassium may rise rapidly requiring an interim dextrose/insulin regimen which, in the antepartum patient, can be followed by dialysis after delivery.

Prior to fetal delivery it is important to optimize placental flow and cardiac output by nursing the patient on her side and maintaining a systolic pressure of 140–160 mmHg. Postdelivery, the patient should not be extubated after section but sedated and returned to the ITU for elective ventilation until the BP has stabilized. This generally takes 24–48 hours.

This patient's condition was complicated by clinical evidence of intra-abdominal haemorrhage. Acute liver rupture is a known but rare complication of the HELLP syndrome. Its management has recently been described by Smith and co-workers. Their recommendation is that hepatic haemorrhage with persistent hypotension unresponsive to blood products should be managed by evacuating the haematoma, packing the damaged liver, and drainage of the operative site. This can be performed immediately after removal of the foetus. More aggressive surgery should be reserved for refractory cases.

KEY POINTS

A diagnosis of HELLP syndrome requires urgent delivery. In addition:

1. Treat bleeding:
   (a) clotting factor replacement – FFP cryoprecipitate;
   (b) platelet infusion – platelets;
   (c) blood volume replacement – blood and colloid or PPF.
2. Regulate therapy by:
   (a) repeated checks of clotting factors and platelets;
   (b) observation of CVP, intra-arterial BP, urine output, and tissue perfusion.

3. Control of BP – once blood volume is replaced the patient is likely to become hypertensive. Monitor intra-arterial BP; maintain at 120/70 to 160/100 by titrated intravenous hydralazine or labetalol. Treat refractory hypertension with additional sublingual nifedipine 10–20 mg, 3–4 hourly.

4. Reduce cerebral irritability. If patient agitation is not resolved by lowering of the BP:
   (a) intravenous magnesium sulphate;
   (b) if concerned about airway or level of agitation – elective intubation and ventilation. Sedate with benzodiazepines.

5. Investigate:
   (a) clotting factors and platelets. Repeat immediately prior to caesarean section;
   (b) ultrasound of abdomen, to assess site of haemorrhage; condition of the liver and foetus to exclude abruptio placenta;
   (c) chest X-ray to exclude pulmonary oedema;
   (d) ECG to exclude any myocardial defect, e.g., cardiomyopathy;
   (e) urinary electrolytes. Urine: sodium < 20 mmol/l; potassium > 50 mmol/l is consistent with acute stress oliguria.

6. Optimize foetal welfare:
   (a) maintain SpO_2 at 98–100%;
   (b) maintain systolic BP > 120, < 160 mmHg; diastolic BP > 70, < 100 mmHg;
   (c) Nurse patient on her side;
   (d) ensure adequate circulating blood volume;
   (e) minimize bleeding diathesis by replacement of clotting factors.

7. Expedite delivery:
   (a) mode of delivery will depend upon the ultrasound findings;
   (b) laparotomy is likely to be required if liver rupture or a subcapsular haematoma is confirmed;
   (c) for management of spontaneous liver rupture during pregnancy, refer to Smith *et al.*;
   (d) if the patient is very ill, consider Caesarean section with post operative ventilation.

8. Monitor:
   (a) CVP; SpO_2; intra-arterial BP; ECG monitor, and fluid balance;
   (b) consider PAOP if pulmonary oedema on chest X-ray or circulating blood volume is in doubt. Perhaps defer insertion until postdelivery.

FURTHER READING

Roberts, J. M. (1995) Magnesium sulphate for pre-eclampsia and eclampsia. N.Engl.J.Med., 333(4), 250–1.

Sibal, B. M. (1990) The HELLP syndrome: much ado about nothing? Am.J.Obstet.Gynaecol., 166, 311–16.

Smith, L. G. Jr., Moise, K. J., Dildy, G. A., and Carpenter, R. J. (1991) Spontaneous rupture of the liver during pregnancy. *Curr.Ther.Obstet.Gynaecol.*, **77**(2), 171–5.

NOTES

8.2 THROMBOCYTOPAENIA

S. J. MACHIN FRCP FRcPath
Professor of Haematology
UCL Hospitals
London

A 35-year-old, caucasian primigravida was admitted as an emergency by her GP when 34 weeks pregnant.

On examination she weighed 104 kg (compared to 85 kg at 12 weeks). She was hypertensive (BP 160/115 mmHg), there was gross oedema of her legs and feet, and urine showed 4+ proteinuria. A diagnosis of pre-eclampsia was made and an emergency Caesarian section was carried out that evening.

Preoperatively her full blood count showed:

Haemoglobin 14.6 g/dl
Platelet count 224 3 109/l
Prothrombin time 14 seconds, control 14 seconds (normal range within 2 seconds of control)
APTT 36 seconds, control 34 seconds (normal range 30–40 seconds)
Thrombin time 14 seconds, control 14 seconds (normal range within 2 seconds of control)
Fibrinogen 3.6 g/l (normal range 1.5–4.0 g/l).

The Caesarian section was uneventful. In particular, there was no excessive bleeding either during or in the immediate postoperative period. A normal, healthy, female, premature infant was born.

On day 1 postoperatively, a coagulation screen showed a falling platelet count (95 × 10^9/l). The patient was unwell and complained of difficulty in breathing.

On day 2 she was oedematous with no urinary output. Haemoglobin was 10.9 g/dl; platelet count 39 × 10^9/l; prothrombin time 18 seconds, control 14 seconds; APTT 51 seconds, control 36 seconds; thrombin time 18 seconds, control 14 seconds; and fibrinogen 1.18 g/l. At this stage she was breathless with evidence of fluid overload, pulmonary oedema, and renal failure. She was transferred to the ICU where she was haemofiltered with standard, unfractionated heparin being given at a dose of 200 u/hour.

The following day (day 3 postdelivery) haemoglobin was 8.6 g/dl; platelet count 24 × 10^9/l; prothrombin time 17 seconds, control 15 seconds; APTT 51 seconds, control 36 seconds, 50/50 mixture 47 seconds; thrombin time 17 seconds, control 14 seconds; fibrinogen 1.41 g/l. A peripheral blood film showed irregularly-contracted red cells, occasionally fragmented red cells, and mild polychromasia. Subsequently, a reticulocyte count was found to be 8.7%. A bone marrow aspirate showed hypercellular haemopoiesis with an increased number of megakaryocytes actively producing platelets. During the day she had started to continuously bleed per vagina and her lochia contained heavy fresh but continuous small clots.

1. COMMENT ON THE DIFFERENTIAL DIAGNOSIS OF THE FALLING PLATELET COUNT AND ASSOCIATED HAEMATOLOGICAL ABNORMALITIES.

2. WHAT FURTHER INVESTIGATIONS SHOULD BE PERFORMED TO SUBSTANTIATE THE DIAGNOSIS?

3. ADVISE ON FUTURE TREATMENT AND MANAGEMENT.

The bone marrow proved that the thrombocytopenia was peripheral and caused by excessive platelet consumption and/or destruction. The differential diagnosis of the peripheral thrombocytopenia with associated polychromatic and fragmented red cells including a raised reticulocyte count with prolongation of the APTT, would have been as follows:

Differential diagnosis

(1) acute disseminated intravascular coagulation (DIC), possibly precipitated by pre-eclampsia;
(2) an immune mediated thrombopenia possibly related to heparin – the so-called heparin-induced thrombocytopenia (HIT syndrome);
(3) The HELLP syndrome in which thrombocytopenia, immediately post-delivery, is associated with red cell haemolysis and elevated liver enzymes;
(4) thrombotic thrombocytopenic purpura (TTP) and/or the haemolytic uraemic syndrome.

DIC

Although the blood film and the reduced platelet count is suggestive of acute DIC, this was unlikely as the thrombin time is only marginally increased and the fibrinogen level is just below the lower limit of normal. For a patient to have this degree of thrombocytopenia, one would expect the thrombin time to be approximately double the control value and the fibrinogen level to be less than 1.0 g/l.

HIT Syndrome

In any patient who is receiving heparin, particularly in the intensive care situation, the possibility of heparin-induced thrombocytopenia with the risk of associated arterial and venous thrombosis must be considered. In patients who have not previously received heparin, the interval between the initiation of heparin therapy and thrombopenia and associated thrombosis is usually about 9 days (range 4–15 days) and decreases to 5 days (range 2–9 days) in patients who have been previously exposed to heparin.

It is believed that heparin-induced antibodies may promote thrombosis through interaction with the endothelial cells. Activated platelets release platelet factor 4 (PF4) from their alpha granules, a protein which is known to bind to heparin. Patients with the HIT syndrome produce antibodies against the heparin PF4 complex which could cause increased platelet activation and induce endothelial cell damage. Recently, an ELISA assay to detect heparin-PF4 complex antibodies has become available and correlates with disease activity and removal of platelets from circulation. Heparin should be discontinued as soon as the diagnosis of HITS is considered, and replaced with other forms of anticoagulation. Low molecular weight heparins are one option, although a more ideal agent is a heparinoid such as ORG 1017, which has a much lower capacity to cross-react with the heparin-induced antibodies. Platelet-associated immunoglobulins were also negative, excluding any immune cause of the thrombopenia.

HELLP

Approximately 10% of pregnancies may be complicated by pre-eclampsia. About 20–25% of patients with pre-eclampsia develop thrombocytopenia and about 10% of patients with pre-eclampsia meet the diagnostic criteria of the HELLP syndrome.

Subsequent biochemical investigation in this patient showed that she did indeed have raised liver enzymes with an AST of 230 iu/l (normal range 0–40); ALT 325 iu/l (normal range 0–35); and a bilirubin of 22 μmol/l (normal range 3–17).

The exact aetiology of thrombocytopenia in this disorder is unclear. However, it is suggested that platelet vascular endothelial cell interactions cause increased platelet consumption. Abnormalities of the coagulation cascade, such as a markedly prolonged prothrombin time, APTT, and a decreased fibrinogen level are quite unusual although mild degrees of excessive thrombin generation do occur. In about 25% of cases the thrombocytopenia only becomes evident after delivery. Very often the pathological microvascular lesions seen in pre-eclampsia and the HELLP syndrome are indistinguishable from those that also occur in TTP. For this reason, plasma exchange with at least 3 litres a day of FFP may be beneficial. The administration of platelet concentrates is not advised as this may precipitate further microvascular thrombosis, causing neurological damage.

TTP

The diagnosis of TTP is often one of exclusion, although frequently these patients have increased circulating levels of the ultra-large, high molecular weight, multimer forms of von Willebrand factor. These are known to substantially increase platelet-induced adhesion and agglutination, leading to platelet consumption and fragmented red cells. It is believed that plasma exchange with FFP removes these pathogenic, ultra-large von Willebrand factor multimers and allows normal processing of the von Willebrand protein to occur, with recovery of the platelet count.

Diagnosis. This patient had a negative heparin-PF4 complex antibody ELISA antibody test, thus excluding heparin-induced thrombopenia as a cause of the low platelet count. She also had a relatively normal thrombin time, prothrombin time, and fibrinogen level, which excludes acute, disseminated, intravascular coagulation as a cause of the red cell fragmentation and the low platelet count. As the patient had developed thrombopenia immediately postdelivery and this was associated with increased liver enzymes, it was diagnostic of the HELLP syndrome. In this patient there were also some similarities with thrombotic thrombocytopenic purpura and it was felt that she had a variant of the HELPP syndrome with associated TTP. Treatment with daily plasma exchange with 3 litres of FFP, continuing haemofiltration, and correction of the fluid overload resulted over the next 4–6 days in normalization of the platelet count and reversal of the acute renal failure and pulmonary oedema. Subsequent analysis of the von Willebrand factor multimer pattern showed increased ultra-large von Willebrand factor fragments prior to the initiation of plasma exchange.

FURTHER READING

Moake, J. L. (1995) Thrombotic thrombocytopenic purpura. *Thrombosis and Haemostasis*, **74**, 240–5.

Sibai, B. M. *et al.* (1993) Maternal morbidity and mortality in 442 pregnancies with haemolysis, elevated liver enzymes, and low platelets (HELLP syndrome). *Am.J.Obstet.Gynaecol.*, **169**, 1000–6.

Wakentin T E. and Kelton, J G. (1990) Heparin and platelets. *Haematol. Oncol.Clin.N.Am.*, **4**, 243–64.

NOTES

8.3 PRE-ECLAMPSIA

D. J. WILLIAMS MRCP

Lecturer in Medicine and Nephrology
Division of Nephrology
UCL Hospitals
London

CASE HISTORY

A 19-year-old primigravida booked in for antenatal care at 14 weeks gestation. BP was 100/65 mmHg and there was no significant past medical history. Her pregnancy progressed uneventfully until 28 weeks when she was admitted from a routine antenatal clinic with a BP of 155/100 mmHg, +++ proteinuria, but no peripheral oedema

INVESTIGATIONS

Biochemistry

Sodium	141 mmol/l	Hb	13.8 g/dl
Potassium	4.5 mmol/l	WCC	5.4×10^9
Urea	6.8 mmol/l	Platelets	116×10^9/l
Creatinine	118 μmol/l	INR	1.2
Urate	360 μmol/l	Thrombin time	15/13
AST	26 iu/l		

She was given methyldopa 250 mg three times a day, which successfully controlled her hypertension, and dexamethasone to accelerate fetal lung maturity. Two days later she developed severe pain in the left side of her abdomen and collapsed. She had a sinus tachycardia; BP 60/30 mmHg; but no vaginal bleeding. Fetal distress was noted on the cardiotocograph. She was given intravenous colloid and had an emergency Caesarean section. At surgery the obstetricians found a large retroplacental haemorrhage that was difficult to stop bleeding. The baby had a poor Apgar score and required ventilation in a special care baby unit. Maternal haematology taken during surgery revealed a prolonged thrombin time (125/14); platelets 28×10^9/; raised fibrin degradation products; and Hb 5.2g/dl. Following surgery she was transferred to ITU. Eighteen hours later she had a grand mal convulsion.

COMMENT ON HER UNDERLYING DISEASE AND FUTURE MANAGEMENT

Pre-eclampsia

This woman had pre-eclampsia, collapsed with placental abruption and DIC, and then had an eclamptic convulsion. Primigravidae are 15 times more likely to develop pre-eclampsia compared to parous women. A rise in diastolic BP > 25 mmHg from a level < 90 mmHg before 20 weeks to > 90 mmHg after 20 weeks defines most cases. Hypertension and an elevated plasma urate (> 0.35 μmol/l at or before 32 weeks, or > 0.40 μmol/l after 32 weeks) are early signs of pre-eclampsia; proteinuria (> 300 mg/24 hours), abnormal liver function, and deranged clotting are late signs. However, none of these features are consistently present. Oedema, which is very common in healthy pregnancy, is no longer used as a discriminatory sign.

Healthy pregnancy is characterized by plasma volume expansion and an elevated glomerular filtration rate (GFR), causing significant reductions in plasma concentrations of urea, creatinine, sodium, liver function tests, and haemoglobin. Pre-eclampsia is a volume-contracted and vaso-constricted state that reverses these changes, causing haemoconcentration, and pushes plasma biochemistry back into normal non-pregnancy ranges, disguising pathology from those unaware of these changes.

Treatment

Controlling moderate hypertension related to pre-eclampsia does not treat the underlying disease, which will progress at an unpredictable rate until baby and placenta are removed.

Low dose aspirin (75 mg daily) has no place in the treatment of pre-eclampsia. However, women who have had severe pre-eclampsia may be protected in future pregnancies if they take low dose aspirin from before 12 weeks gestation to about 30 weeks.

Placental abruption and DIC

The only way to halt progression of this disease is by termination of the pregnancy. Until the patient can be taken to the operating theatre, initial resuscitation is aimed at treatment of hypovolaemic shock using artificial colloids, or crystalloids if colloid is not available. Dextrans should be avoided as they interfere with platelet function. As soon as possible she should be given FFP (contains clotting factors) and cross-matched blood. Un-crossmatched group specific blood (her blood group should be known if ante-natal care is at this hospital) is a life-saving option if there are delays in receiving cross-matched blood. These manoeuvres, along with contraction of the emptied uterus, should be enough to stop bleeding.

Transfusion of fresh platelets is controversial. It has been suggested that they act as fuel for DIC but, if bleeding persists and platelets are less than $20 \times 10^9/l$, transfusion of fresh platelets is sensible. Further controversy surrounds the use of anticoagulants, but at present the balance of argument favours avoiding them.

Regional anaesthesia for surgery should be avoided due to the bleeding risk and because vasodilatation of lower limb vasculature will aggravate hypotension. Fluid replacement needs to be monitored by a central venous line and urinary catheter.

Eclampsia

Although pre-eclampsia cannot improve until baby and placenta are delivered, the disease process can still evolve for up to a week postpartum. In this patient, before diagnosing eclampsia, a convulsion secondary to hypotension and hypoxia must be excluded. A cerebral bleed secondary to DIC is also possible, and once the patient is stable, can be excluded by a CT scan. Immediate management of the convulsion must ensure a clear airway and oxygen administration. The convulsion should be stopped with diazemuls 10 mg as an i.v. bolus, followed 1–2 minutes later by another 10 mg.

Until recently, controversy has surrounded the choice of agent that best prevents further eclamptic convulsions. Now, evidence from the Collaborative Eclampsia Trial firmly places magnesium sulphate, rather than phenytoin or diazemuls, as the agent of choice to prevent recurrent convulsions. Magnesium sulphate is not an anticonvulsant, and unlike diazemuls, will not stop a convulsion. Having first controlled a convulsion, magnesium sulphate 4 g should be given intravenously over 5 minutes as a loading dose, followed by an infusion of 1 g/hour for 24 hours. If convulsions recur then another 2 g i.v. bolus should be given over 5 minutes. It is usually not necessary to measure magnesium levels. Prophylactic magnesium sulphate for women with pre-eclampsia (i.e. those who have not yet had a convulsion) remains of unproven benefit.

KEY POINTS

1. Controlling moderate hypertension related to pre-eclampsia does not treat the underlying disease.
2. Pre-eclampsia can progress for up to a week postpartum.
3. Treatment of DIC involves: (i) removal of the initiating event, e.g. placental abruption; and (ii) support of the circulation with colloid, lost blood products, and clotting factors.
4. Magnesium sulphate is the best drug for prevention of recurrent eclamptic convulsions.

FURTHER READING

The Eclampsia Trial Collaborative Group. (1995) Which anticonvulsant for women with eclampsia? Evidence from the Collaborative Eclampsia Trial. *Lancet*, 345, 1455–63.

Further readinMacGillivray, I. (1959) Some observations on the incidence of pre-eclampsia. J.Obstet.Gynaecol.British Commonwealth, 65, 536–9.

Redman, C. W. G. and Jeffries, M. (1988) Revised definition of pre-eclampsia. *Lancet* (i) 809, 812.

I. MURDOCH D.CH. MRCP
Consultant Paediatrician
Paediatric ICU
Guys Hospital
London

CASE HISTORY

A 20-month-old child arrived in A&E, collapsed with a florid purpuric rash. He was febrile (central temperature 39.1°C) but had cold, dusky peripheries. Initial assessment revealed a BP of 45/30 mmHg; pulse 150/min; capillary refill time > 3 seconds. Respirations were shallow at a rate of 50/min. He was rousable but agitated and did not respond to his parents.

INVESTIGATIONS

Biochemistry

Sodium	145 mmol/l
Potassium	3.7 mmol/l
Chloride	104 mmol/l
Urea	11.9 mmol/l
Creatinine	130 μmol/l
Glucose	10.2 mmol/
Calcium	1.6 mmol/l
Magnesium	0.55 mmol/l

Hb	10.5g/dl
WCC	2.1×10^9/l
Platelets	28×10^9/l
INR	4.52
Fibrinogen	1.2g/l

pH	7.05
$PaCO_2$	3.2 kPa
$PaCO_2$	8.6 kPa
HCO_3	9.4 mmol/l
BE	−12 mmols/l
Serum lactate	9.4 mmol/l

DISCUSS MANAGEMENT OF THIS PATIENT

This child has meningococcal septicaemia, complicated by DIC and purpura fulminans. Meningitis may coexist but does not influence his immediate management. He is shocked with biochemical evidence of severe tissue hypoxia. A variable level of consciousness and respiratory symptoms are indications for intubation and ventilation. Vascular access is required. Central venous cannulation is preferred but resuscitation can be adequately performed with peripheral lines or intraosseous needles. A urinary catheter should be sited. Blood cultures are drawn and antibiotics administered (cefotaxime 200 mg/kg/day).

Hypovolaemia should be corrected with repeated 10–20 ml aliquots of colloid. Underestimation of the volume required to attain fluid replacement is common. Capillary leak and right ventricular dysfunction may mean infusion of 50–100 ml/kg of fluid before adequate stabilization is achieved. CVP should be maintained at levels normally considered supranormal. Hypotension, despite aggressive fluid replacement, is an indication for inotropic support (dopamine/dobutamine 5–20 mcg/kg/min, or adrenaline 0.1–10 mcg/kg/min). Peripheral perfusion may be improved utilizing prostacyclin 5–20 ng/kg/min in those patients in whom its hypotensive effects are not destabilizing. Sodium bicarbonate is employed to reduce the level of acidosis if the pH falls below 7.1. Crystalloid maintenance replacement is restricted to 50% of normal requirement.

DIC is invariable in the shocked meningococcaemic patient. Gross coagulation dysfunction results in microvascular thrombosis with the appearance of a purpuric rash. FFP and platelets have been the mainstays of therapy for this complication. However, this treatment is sub-optimal following discovery of the role of proteins C and S and antithrombin III in severe DIC. FFP is a poor source of protein C and effective replacement is easier with concentrates. Vitamin K, upon which the production of numerous clotting factors (including proteins C and S) are dependent, should be administered. Seeking haematological advice will clarify treatment.

Hypocalcaemia and hypomagnesaemia occur with such frequency that their presence should be assumed and measures taken to rectify a deficit. This child already has multi-organ failure at the time of admission. The failure of other organ systems and a deterioration in function of those already involved should be anticipated and managed aggressively.

KEY POINTS

1. The intraosseous route is effective for the administration of the emergency drugs and volume replacement.
2. Initial stabilization may involve colloid infusions totalling 50–100 ml/kg. First day volume replacement may be twice this amount. Be aggressive!

FURTHER READING

Leclerc, F. *et al.* (1992) Protein C and S deficiency in severe infectious purpura of children: a collaborative study of 40 cases. *Int.Care Med.*, **18**, 202–5.

Mercier, J. C., Beaufils, F. and Hartmann, J. F. (1988) Hemodynamic patterns of meningococcal shock in children. *Crit. Care Med.*, **16**, 27–33.

Orlowski J. P., Porembka, D. T., Gallagher, J. M., *et al.* (1990) Comparison study of Intraosseous, central intravenous, and peripheral intravenous infusions of emergency drugs. *Am.J.Dis.Child*, **144**:112–7.

NOTES

8.5 CROUP

D. J. MACRAE FRCA
Consultant in Paediatric Intensive Care
Great Ormond Street Children's Hospital
London

CASE HISTORY

A two-year-old child presented with a 3-day history of coryzal symptoms. Until that morning her symptoms had apparently been well-palliated with regular administration of paracetamol suspension, and she had continued to eat and drink. However, her parents were awoken at 5am by her coughing, and on the advice of their GP, took the child to the emergency department.

On examination the child had a respiratory rate of 40/min and an axillary temperature of 38.2°C. High-pitched inspiratory stridor and harsh coughing episodes were noted during the examination, which was conducted with the child sitting on her mother's lap. Intercostal and sternal recession were also evident and the child appeared sleepy in between coughing episodes.

WHAT IS THE LIKELY DIAGNOSIS? DESCRIBE YOUR INITIAL ASSESSMENT AND MANAGEMENT OF THE CHILD

Differential diagnosis. This child had a prodromal illness and now presents with cough and signs of upper-airway obstruction.

Acute laryngotracheobronchitis ('croup') typically presents in children aged 6 months to 3 years. The onset of stridor, which is the result of subglottic oedema, is preceded by symptoms of a mild, respiratory viral infection. Barking cough is a prominent feature of croup, which is usually the result of parainfluenza virus, respiratory syncytial virus, or adenovirus infection. Spasmodic allergic croup, bacterial tracheitis, foreign body aspiration, and acute epiglottitis should be considered in the differential diagnosis.

Assessment and management. This child has severe upper-airway obstruction, is tiring, and is at risk of sustaining a respiratory arrest if the airway obstruction is not relieved. Attempts at examining the throat, and painful procedures such as venepuncture and venous cannulation may precipitate complete airway obstruction and should be avoided until the airway is secure.

The definitive management of acute upper airway obstruction is tracheal intubation facilitated by oxygen–halothane inhalational anaesthesia. This should be undertaken by an experienced anaesthetist in the ICU or emergency department. There is no place for tracheostomy in the routine management of croup.

Nebulized adrenaline (2.5 ml of 1: 1000 solution) may temporarily improve a child's airway by vasoconstricting inflamed mucosal surfaces. Nebulized adrenaline can be administered prior to induction of anaesthesia for intubation. It may also be used in less severe cases in an attempt to improve the airway and avoid the need for intubation. Conservative management with adrenaline nebulizers should only be considered if the child can be monitored in a high-dependency unit. Children requiring more than three doses in 12 hours and those whose response is transient, require intubation.

Airway obstruction in croup is subglottic and laryngoscopy is usually straightforward. An ETT 0.5 or 1.0 mm internal diameter (ID) smaller than the age-appropriate size should be used. Secretions are copious in viral croup. There is a considerable danger of tube occlusion from secretions if they cannot be cleared easily, and for this reason very small tubes (more than 1.0 mm below age-appropriate size, or tubes < 3.0 mm ID) should not be used.

Steroids are of proven value in intubated patients with croup and should be administered until 24 hours after extubation. The ETT must be retained by meticulous fixation, respiratory gases humidified, and secretions aspirated regularly. Some paediatric ICUs manage intubated children with croup without sedation, using distraction from toys or carers to prevent anxiety. Other units fully sedate such children, although this in turn may necessitate ventilation.

Extubation is usually undertaken after 5–7 days or whenever an air leak is audible around the ET when 25–30 cm water pressure is applied. The child is extubated in routine fashion, with anaesthetist and reintubation facilities to hand should the extubation fail.

KEY POINTS

1. Prednisolone 1 mg/kg 8–12 hourly has been shown to reduce the duration of intubation in infants with croup.
2. Always use an ETT 0.5–1.0 mm smaller than usual when intubating patients with croup.

FURTHER READING

Ackerman, V. L. and Harris, J. M. (1992) Specific diseases of the respiratory system: upper airway. In (ed. B. P. Furhman and J. J. Zimmerman) *Pediatric Critical Care*. Mosby Year Book, St Louis.

Backofen, J. E. and Rogers, M. C. (1992) Upper airway disease. In (ed. M. C. Rogers) *Textbook of pediatric intensive care*, 2nd edn, Williams Wilkins, Baltimore.

NOTES

8.6 RESPIRATORY FAILURE IN THE INFANT

M. Peters MRCP
Senior Registrar

R. C. Tasker FRCP
Consultant Physician
Intensive Care Unit
Great Ormond Street Children's Hospital
London

CASE HISTORY

A 4 month-old Asian infant was admitted from the general paediatric ward. She had been an inpatient for 3 days with a respiratory illness, but was now requiring increasing oxygen supplementation and looked tired.

EXAMINATION FINDINGS

Weight 3.5 kg; temp 37°C; respiratory rate 80/min; heart rate 175/min; BP 60/40 mmHg; SpO_2 82% (70% head box oxygen); palpable 2cm liver edge.

INVESTIGATIONS

Hb	6.7 g/dl
WCC	$7.3 \times 10^9/l$ (neutrophils 6.7, lymph 0.3)
Platelets	$197 \times 10^9/l$
Electrolytes	normal
Chest X-ray:	diffuse airspace shadowing throughout both lung fields; low volume lungs

WHAT IS THE DIFFERENTIAL DIAGNOSIS?

This child has a diffusely abnormal chest X-ray. Infective causes must be considered first. Respiratory syncytial virus pneumonitis would be possible in the winter months though a uniformly abnormal chest X-ray is unusual. Cardiogenic pulmonary oedema from congenital heart disease may present in this way with an obstructive lesion (aortic stenosis, coarctation) though careful clinical examination can exclude many such cases. Obstructed, anomalous, pulmonary venous drainage would need to be excluded by expert echocardiographic examination.

This child has a congenital, severe, combined immunodeficiency and PCP. Pointers to this diagnosis are the poor growth (3.5 kg at 4 months); low haemoglobin, suggesting chronic illness; and particularly, the very abnormal low lymphocyte count (a detailed family history is also often informative). Human immunodeficiency virus (HIV) infection is possible but very uncommon in the Asian population.

WHAT SIMPLE DIAGNOSTIC INVESTIGATIONS WOULD YOU PERFORM?

A simple diagnostic investigation for respiratory viruses and PCP is the examination of secretions collected by nasopharyngeal aspiration with immunoflouresence.

OUTLINE INITIAL RESUSCITATION AND FURTHER MANAGEMENT

Initial resuscitation requires intubation and ventilation. This child will require a size 4 ETT. PCV with permissive hypercapnia ($PaCO_2$ 7–8.5 kPa and pH $>$ 7.25) with high PEEP and inverse inspired:expired ratio (if required) should be used to limit ventilator-induced secondary lung injury while maximizing lung volume. Intravenous fluid intake should be restricted to 60 ml/kg/24 hours given as 10% dextrose + 0.18% saline initially, but may be reduced further.

Specific therapy with co-trimoxazole should be commenced and consideration given to the possible coexistence of other infection (especially mycobacterial or cytomegalovirus) before the addition of steroid therapy. Transfusion of unirradiated blood to such a child carries the small but potentially fatal risk of transfusional graft vs host disease.

WHAT STEPS WOULD YOU CONSIDER IN THE EVENT OF PROGRESSIVE RESPIRATORY FAILURE?

In the face of continued deterioration of respiratory function alternative strategies include the use of high frequency oscillatory ventilation, surfactant therapy, and inhaled nitric oxide.

This child would not currently be considered for extracorporeal membrane oxygenation because of the nature of the underlying condition.

KEY POINTS

1. Age-specific normal ranges for weight, cardiovascular parameters, respiratory rate, and ETT size are essential knowledge (see Table 2).
2. The severity of secondary, ventilator-induced lung injury (oxygen toxicity, volutrauma, or barotrauma) may be limited by the use of permissive hypercarbia in association with strategies to maintain mean airway pressure (and hence lung volume) by the use of PEEP and inverse-ratio ventilation.
3. Even in the absence of clinical fluid overload, gas exchange may be improved by fluid restriction.

Table 2 is simplified for ease of use but some simple rules can be used as a guide when this is not available, e.g.:

Table 1

- ETT size (diameter mm) = (age/4) + 4
- length (to lips cm) = (age/2) + 12
- respiratory rate = 40 − age in years
- Weight (kg) = (age + 4) × 2.

Table 2 Normal values by age for weight (kg), ETT diameter (mm), respiratory rate (breath/min, heart rate (beats/min), and blood pressure (mmHg).

Age	Weight	ETT size	Respiratory rate	Heart rate	BP
Premature infant	0.5–2.5	2.0–3.0	60	120	40–60 (systolic)
Term infant	3.5	3.5	40	120	75/50
1–6 months	4–7	3.5–4.0	40	140	80/50
6–12 months	7–10	4.0	40	130	90/65
12–24 months	10–12	3.0–5.0	38	120	95/65
2–6 years	12–20	4.5–5.5	34–38	108	100/60

FURTHER READING

Advanced paediatric life support; the practical approach. BMJ Publishing Group, London.

Arnold, R., *et al.* (1994) Prospective, randomized comparison of HFOV and conventional mechanical ventilation in pediatric respiratory failure. *Crit.Care Med.*, 22, 486–91.

Shuster, D. P. (1995) Fluid management in ARDS: 'Keep them dry or does it matter?' *Int. Care Med.*, 21, 101–2.

Part 9 Ethics

9.1 Withdrawal of treatment

S. L. COHEN FRCP
Consultant Physician
Intensive Care Unit
UCL Hospitals
London

CASE HISTORY

A 22-year-old female patient, married with a young child, was diagnosed as having acute leukaemia. She developed respiratory and renal failure following bone marrow transplantation. She was leucopenic and thrombocytopenic. The haematologists considered both conditions were reversible and she was transferred to the ICU for ventilation and haemofiltration.

Her condition steadily deteriorated. Sepsis and ARDS developed but no organisms were found. She had been on positive pressure ventilation for ARDS for 12 days with 100% oxygen, and had been haemofiltered for 8 days. There were no signs of improvement. In the opinion of the staff there was no hope of recovery.

HOW WOULD YOU ARRIVE AT A DECISION TO WITHDRAW THERAPY?

The first responsibility of the intensive care clinician is to ensure that the medical facts are verified, that the patient has been given optimal treatment, and every chance to recover. In a case like this it is essential to review the care strategy regularly. The question of withdrawal of intensive care support is a very contentious one and is exceptionally difficult. A protocol has been developed in our own unit for withdrawal of life support.

1. The consultant in charge must be sure, as far as clinically possible, that there is no reasonable hope that the patient can survive and that treatment will not benefit the patient.
2. There must be general consensus of agreement among the ITU and primary team staff that death is inevitable. This opinion will be reached after consultations and case conferences if necessary. The deliberations must be recorded in the notes.
3. A second consultant must agree. If the admitting consultant is not available, a second ITU consultant should be involved.
4. The patient's views, if known, should be sought, e.g. from living will or durable power of attorney or by discussion with the patient's family and friends. The patient's known views should be respected. All these procedures must be recorded in notes. A living will which refuses medical treatment is binding, provided it was made by a patient when competent and was clearly intended by the patient to apply to the prevailing situation.
5. The family, partners, or carers must be fully and frequently informed of the decision-making process and they must assent.
6. All these procedures must be recorded in the notes and the patient's condition reviewed at regular intervals. A treatment plan must be defined. It must be stressed that care continues.
7. Staff who have objections to the change of emphasis in care should be allowed not to participate.
8. Care continues, but the aim of treatment is altered towards allowing the patient as peaceful and dignified a death as possible.

IF WITHDRAWAL WAS AGREED, HOW WOULD YOU MANAGE THIS SITUATION?

1. Withdrawal of treatment measures such as antibiotics, drugs to support BP, steroids, blood products, haemofiltration or dialysis.
2. Ventilator management. Continue ventilation for comfort – reduce unnecessarily high oxygen concentrations. If the patient can breathe comfortably and is able to maintain an airway, the ETT should be removed.

3. Continue all treatment required for the patient's comfort e.g. sedation, analgesia, and hydration.

KEY POINTS

1. The decision to allow a patient to die should be a consensus one and should be regularly reviewed.
2. The patient's known wishes must be respected.
3. The family, partners, and carers should be in agreement with the plan.

FURTHER READING

Cohen, S. L. (1993) *Whose life is it anyhow*. Intensive care – when to stop, pp. 40–6. Robson Books, London.

(1993) *Medical ethics today, its practice and philosophy*. Withdrawing Treatment, pp 170–171. BMA, London.

Index